"Deep brain stimulation has revolutionized our approach to the treatment of Parkinson's disease, dystonia and tremor. The book 'DBS: A Patient Guide to Deep Brain Stimulation' by the team of Monique Giroux MD and Sierra Farris PA-C offers patients and caregivers a practical guide to deep brain stimulation that is long overdue. It addresses practical everyday questions that both patients and physicians alike will find extremely helpful covering a broad array of topics related to DBS. The book is highly informative, thorough and written at a level that is easy to understand. This book is a must for patients considering DBS and for physicians who take care of patients who may be candidates for DBS."

-Jerrold L Vitek MD, PhD, McKnight Professor and Head, Director, Neuromodulation Research Center, Department of Neurology, University of Minnesota School of Medicine

"The authors are respected clinicians who are experienced with all facets of the management of Parkinson's disease. They have written a very sophisticated and complete handbook for patients who are considering or have already undergone Deep Brain Stimulation. This book will be essential for patients who are looking for a more in-depth resource about a complex topic in Parkinson's disease management."

-Melanie Brandabur MD, Clinic Director, Parkinson's Institute and Clinical Center, Sunnyvale, CA

"I liked the six main goals in managing the DBS device. It helps the programmer and patients to clarify and develop similar goals of programming so patients can have realistic expectations. The book contains the best explanation of programming and stimulation adjustments that I've ever read. This topic is abstract and difficult for the unscientific mind to grasp. Thanks for making it understandable. My favorite section -Symptoms and Expectations Exercise, helps explain to patients how to concretely identify their expectations about DBS. Great explanation of targeting, head frame, frameless, bilateral staged, bilateral simultaneous, burr hole, nerve cell recording, and testing."

-Kate Kelsall, person living with DBS; Co-founder The Bionic Brigade Denver DBS Support Group and Co-Founder and President of DBS Voices of the Rockies

DBS

A Patient Guide to Deep Brain Stimulation

DEDICATION

This book is dedicated to our patients.

I am only one, but still I am one. I cannot do everything, but still I can do something; and because I cannot do everything, I will not refuse to do something that I can do.
-Helen Keller

ACKNOWLEDGMENTS

The authors wish to acknowledge and thank our patients. Their courage and strength have been a source of inspiration. Special thanks to Jill Ater, Edna Ball, Alice Cleeton, Dean Crumpacker, Michael Erb, Michael Kinsley, and Gayle Schendzielos whose message and stories remind us of the power of hope. We also wish to thank Kate Kelsall, MSW for an expedited review of a partial manuscript and thoughtful comments.

We extend our appreciation to Ingrid McGruder for the energy, dedication and compassion she brings to work every day.

A special thank you to Jerrold Vitek, MD, PhD for his ongoing mentorship and friendship throughout the years.

DBS

A Patient Guide to Deep Brain Stimulation

Sierra M. Farris, MA, MPAS, PA-C
Director Deep Brain Stimulation Services
Movement & Neuroperformance Center Colorado
Staff at Swedish Hospital, Englewood Colorado
www.dbsprogrammer.com

Monique L. Giroux, MD
Medical Director and CEO
Movement & Neuroperformance Center Colorado
Medical Director of Movement Disorders & DBS Program at Swedish Hospital, Englewood Colorado
Medical Director of Northwest Parkinson's Foundation, Seattle Washington
www.drgiroux.com

First Edition 2013

Movement & Neuroperformance Center Colorado, P.C.
499 E. Hampden Avenue, Suite 250 Englewood, Colorado 80113
Phone 303-781-0511; Fax 303-781-0517
www.centerformovement.org

Disclaimer: The content represents the opinions and experience of the authors and is meant to be used for educational purposes only. This information should not be considered a substitute for medical professional advice or care. This book does not replace the medical advice of your physician. Readers should always discuss any information, questions or treatments with their medical providers. The authors do not accept any responsibility for liability, loss, risk or complications that may be claimed or incurred as a consequence of the content in this book.

ISBN-13: 978-1491283158
ISBN-10: 1491283157

CONTENTS

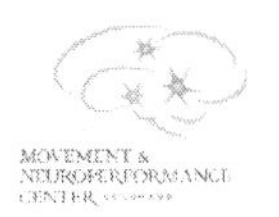

FORWARD

Parkinson's disease is a life altering diagnosis for those directly affected, their families and their care-partners. For most, after an initial phase of disbelief and misunderstanding, the symptoms become a way of life. None of us would choose Parkinson's. But, once chosen by Parkinson's, the decision clearly becomes one of choice between inaction, worsening symptoms and depression or acknowledgement, education, support and empowerment to move forward.

I am personally thrilled this book is being published. I am even more heartened by your decision to educate yourself and those around you with the latest information on the potential options to ameliorate your symptoms and live the best life possible. And, while ultimately, your best treatment decisions will be made between you and your neurologist or movement disorder specialist, I applaud you for taking the lead on this journey to know the advantages and the side effects of Deep Brain Stimulation. As Francis Bacon, Thomas Jefferson and others have suggested, k*nowledge is power. This book will certainly grant you the power of knowledge at a time when control and the power of movement might evade you.*

Monique Giroux, MD and Sierra Farris, PAC have long been considered thought leaders in the movement disorders field with their empathic patient centered approach to care. Their work at the Northwest Parkinson's Foundation and directly with their patients has always centered on one simple postulate—improve the quality of life of persons with Parkinson's. As members of the NWPF Board of Directors for many years, Dr. Giroux and Sierra helped foster a legion of empowered patients, committed volunteers, practitioners and care-partners dedicated to that purpose. Yesterday, today and tomorrow, until the cure is uncovered, the authors and Northwest Parkinson's Foundation will work tirelessly in the pursuit of improving the quality of life of persons with Parkinson's.

The book you hold will do more than help you decide your best treatment pathway. Dr. Giroux and Sierra share their knowledge with you, and offer a powerful message urging you and your family to become an active participant in your care to ultimately gain a greater quality of life regardless of the pathway you choose. And, once upon that path, this book and the Northwest Parkinson's Foundation will help guide you to obtain the most you can from the treatment you have chosen.

--Steve Wright, Executive Director Northwest Parkinson's Foundation, Seattle Washington

DBS

A Patient Guide to Deep Brain Stimulation

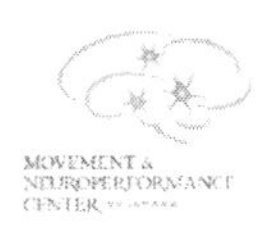

1 OVERVIEW OF DEEP BRAIN STIMULATION

"DBS changed my life. Or rather, it didn't change my life--it allowed me to stay more or less the same. Since my surgery in 2006, there has been no visible change in my condition or symptoms. Previously, I was declining a bit, but a noticeable bit, each year. I know people who have not had such a successful outcome, but more people who have. 'Brain surgery' is scary, but DBS surgery was nowhere near as unpleasant as I expected. True, I've had better days. But most of them have been since the operation."

-Michael Kinsley

Introduction

Whether you already have deep brain stimulation (DBS) or just want to learn more, this patient guide is for you. We share insights from over a decade of experience treating people with DBS in a holistic movement disorders clinic. We pass this information on with one goal in mind, to inspire you to take an active role in your care and offer simple tools to help you along the way to live your best with DBS.

If you are new to DBS, the decision to undergo surgery can be a difficult one. If you already have DBS, you will want to stay up-to-date over the years. Armed with practical and useful information compiled by DBS experts, you will have the insight you need to guide DBS related treatment decisions. But information is not enough.

We urge you to become an engaged partner in your care. *"An engaged patient is an informed and empowered patient."* Throughout this book you will find suggestions and worksheets to help you understand how DBS therapy will work for you, provide guidance when you need to make treatment decisions and offer tips to minimize problems while living with DBS. We encourage you to download the worksheets from our companion website DBSGUIDE.COM and complete the self-assessment exercises. By sharing the results with your medical team, you are guiding your care with a focus on your personal needs and preferences.

Visit DBSGUIDE.COM to download and print additional copies of the worksheets and assessment tools found in this book.

What is deep brain stimulation?

Deep brain stimulation (DBS) is a Food and Drug Administration (FDA) approved surgical treatment for medical conditions including Parkinson's disease (PD), tremor and dystonia. Prior to DBS, surgical treatment for tremor and PD included lesion surgery called thalamotomy and pallidotomy. Lesion surgery involves the permanent destruction of brain cells in specific brain regions. DBS is a significant advance since unlike lesion surgery, DBS is reversible (the hardware can be removed), brain tissue damage is minimized and the therapy is customized to each patient and their symptoms.

The surgical procedure involves implanting tiny wire(s) into the brain. The wires have four small electrodes that deliver customized continuous electrical impulses to regions deep in the brain. A neurostimulator (also called battery or pulse generator) provides the power to send the impulses along the wire. The neurostimulator is implanted outside the brain under the collarbone.

DBS Hardware Components

Currently, the only U.S. Food and Drug Administration (FDA) approved DBS hardware system is manufactured by Medtronic Inc. The (Medtronic) hardware system includes the following components:

Lead Wire – The lead wire is implanted directly into the brain through a small hole made in the skull that is about the size of a dime. At the end of the wire are four tiny electrode bands (shown on right) that are spaced vertically and numbered 0, 1, 2, 3. Length of each electrode is 1.5 millimeters.

Plastic Cap – A small plastic ring is secured with tiny screws and the attached cap permanently covers the hole in the skull and secures the wire.

Extension Wire – An extension wire connects the lead wire in the brain to the neurostimulator battery that is outside the brain.

Practical Tips: The wires are insulated. When intact, energy flowing along the wire is not felt. If the wire or insulation is damaged, energy can flow into adjacent tissue resulting in tingling, heat or electrical sensations in that area. Report this to your provider.

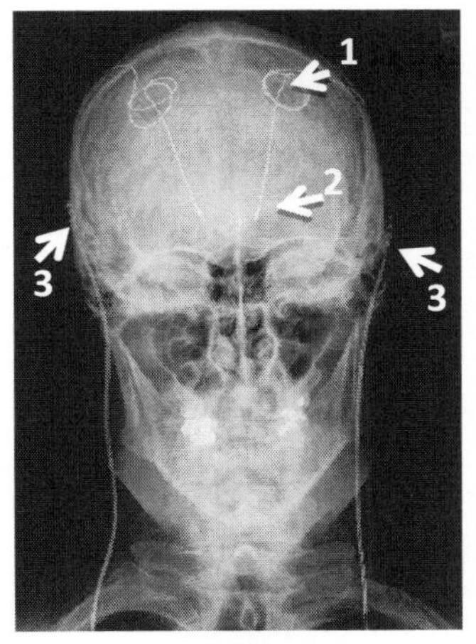

X-Rays of the implanted system. The skull x-ray (upper left) shows the lead wires positioned deep in the brain. The wires enter the brain through a hole in the skull (#1) and are anchored with a plastic cap not visible on x-ray. The excess wire is coiled near the cap. The tip of the wire is the location of the stimulating electrodes (#2). The connection between the lead wire and extension wire is noted on each side of the head just above the ear (#3). The x-ray illustrates bilateral implants with an extension wire connecting to a neurostimulator on each side of the chest.

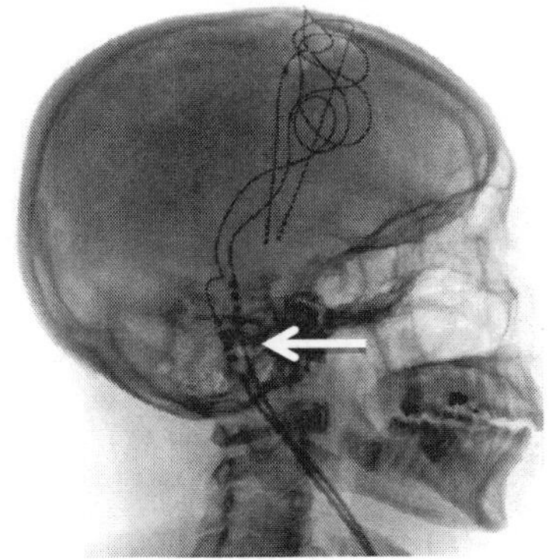

The x-ray (left) shows a side view of the skull. Note the large coils of extra wire. The excess wire is difficult to feel which reinforces the warning to avoid head massage, scalp acupuncture and laser surgery. The connection between the lead wire and the extension wire is highlighted by the white arrow. The connection can be felt as a lump under the skin is typically is a sensitive area for several weeks after DBS surgery.

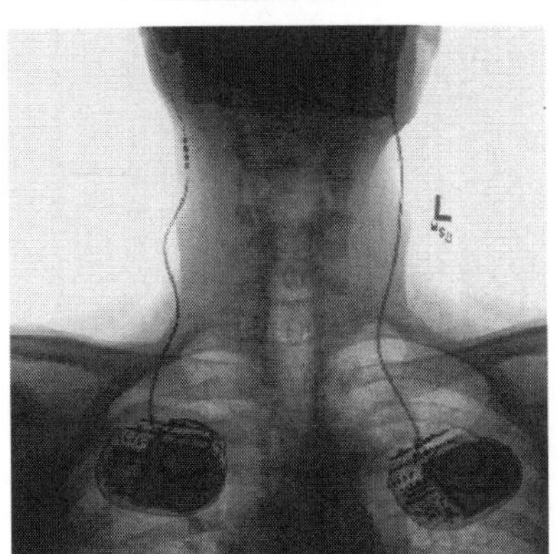

The x-ray (bottom left) shows the extension wire tunnel from the head to the chest. The neurostimulator is typically implanted under the collarbone. All hardware components are implanted under the skin. Once all hardware components are connected, stimulation can be applied. Any disruption in the hardware system will limit or prohibit the flow of electricity to the brain. Electricity leakage into the tissue can be felt as warmth, tingling, minor shock sensations or buzzing that can be intermittent or constant depending on the wire damage.

Neurostimulator Options

Medtronic manufactured neurostimulators are the most common implanted systems for DBS worldwide. There are currently three FDA approved models available for DBS. Deciding which neurostimulator is right for you will depend on factors such as whether stimulation is needed on one or both sides of the brain, stimulation intensity, personal lifestyle preferences and insurance coverage. The neurostimulators have a microchip that stores names, diagnosis, surgery date, physician and most recent stimulation settings.

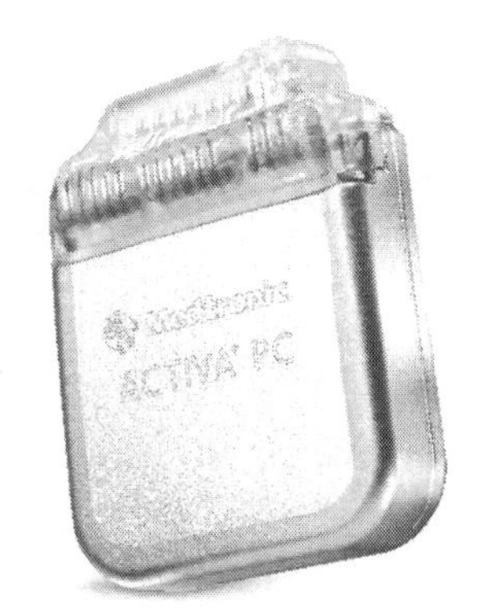

Activa® PC – The PC neurostimulator is a dual channel battery that provides stimulation for two lead wires (when the left and right brain are implanted). The PC is an option when stimulation is needed for both sides of the body. The PC lasts 2 to 4 years depending on stimulation intensity.

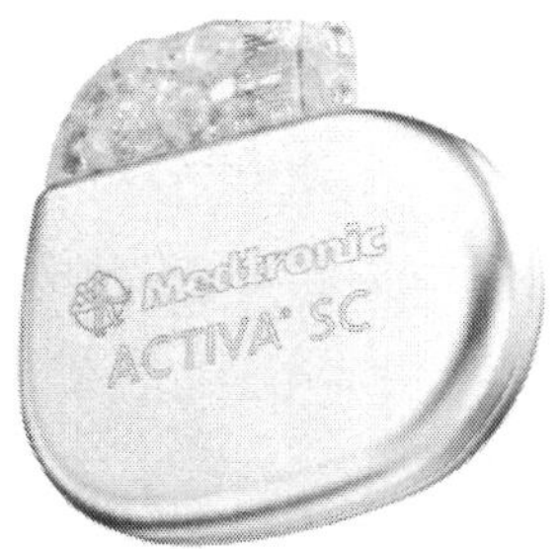

Activa® SC – The SC neurostimulator is a single channel battery that provides stimulation for one lead wire. The SC is smaller and a common choice when one side of the brain is implanted. The SC has the same features as the PC and generally lasts 3 to 5 years depending on stimulation intensity.

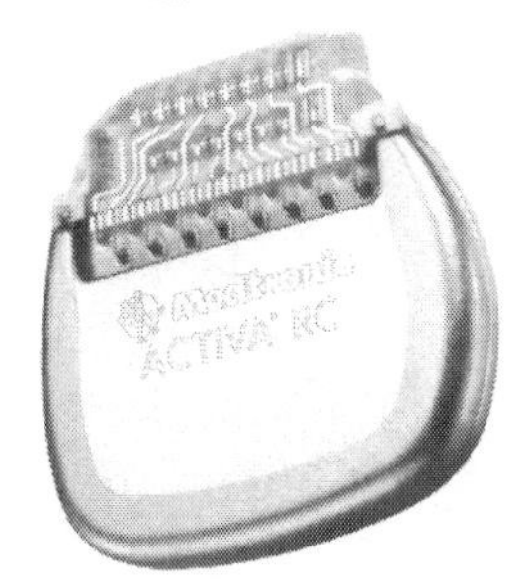

Activa® RC – The RC is a re-chargeable dual channel neurostimulator that requires recharging typically every one to two weeks depending on stimulation intensity. The RC will last 9 years regardless of stimulation intensity and may be beneficial for conditions (such as dystonia) that may require high settings that place more demand on the neurostimulator. The RC reduces the frequency of replacement surgery but requires the commitment to recharge.

(Images of Medtronic, Inc. Activa components and hardware are reprinted with the permission of Medtronic, Inc. © 2013)

Practical Tips: Discuss battery options during your consultation for surgery. Be sure to discuss where the battery will be implanted (i.e., left or right upper chest).

Patient Programmer: a patient programmer (on right) allows you to check whether the stimulation is *on* or *off*, and *battery status*. The patient programmer also allows you to make pre-determined stimulation changes at home if your healthcare provider has activated this feature. You can only adjust stimulation settings pre-set by your healthcare provider during your medical appointment. Not everyone will need to make stimulation changes but this feature is helpful to adjust stimulation at home.

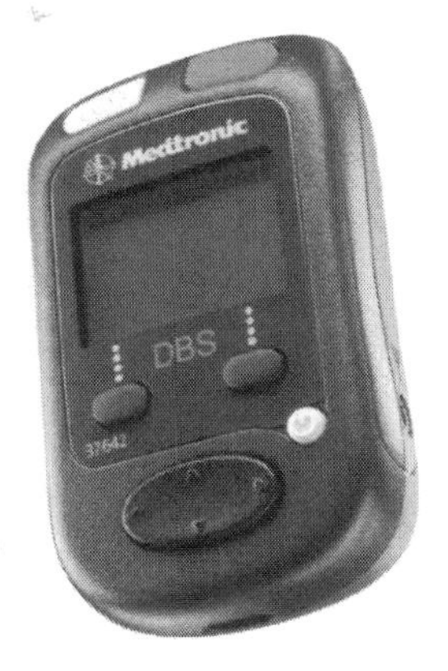

Physician Programmer Device: Stimulation is adjusted using a small handheld device. Using a touch screen, signals are sent along a cable to the neurostimulator and stimulation settings are saved to the neurostimulator. The neurostimulator also saves the four most recent stimulation visits for later reference.

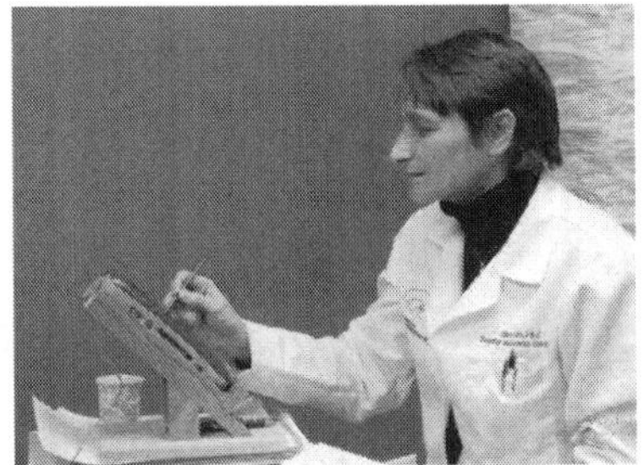

How does DBS work?

Exactly how DBS improves symptoms associated with Parkinson's disease, tremor or dystonia is unknown. We do know that neurons in specific brain regions emit abnormal electrical firing patterns in each of these conditions. These abnormal firing patterns are associated with the motor symptoms of the disease. The DBS electrodes are implanted into these brain areas and appropriate application of stimulation works to restore normal signal patterns allowing for improved movement patterns and improved muscle tone.

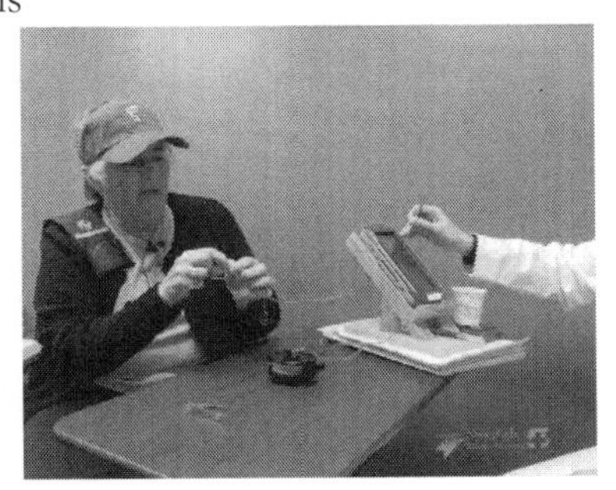

Stimulation is adjustable and the effects are reversible. For example, specific stimulation parameters (voltage, frequency, pulse width) are set by your programmer, depending on location of the electrodes, to achieve motor benefit and avoid stimulation side effects. If stimulation is turned off, the effect will disappear and symptoms will usually return.

IT IS IMPORTANT TO NOTE THAT DBS IS NOT A CURE. Deep brain stimulation can improve very specific movement symptoms and excessive muscle tone with accurate electrode placement and appropriately applied stimulation. It is very important to understand which symptoms should improve since not all movement problems respond to DBS. Knowing how DBS can help will give you specific talking points to discuss with your doctor whether you are considering DBS or have been living with DBS. The next section(s) will describe the different brain regions implanted and specific symptoms that can be improved with each of these brain targets.

Three Brain Targets

Parkinson's disease, tremor and dystonia cause symptoms of excessive muscle tone, tremor, slowness, change in coordination, walking, posture and balance problems. The brain regions selected for these conditions include the subthalamic nucleus (STN), globus pallidus interna (GPi) and thalamus (specific region of thalamus is the ventralis intermedialis or Vim) shown in the figure. Each of these brain targets are part of a complex and interrelated connection of nerve cells called the basal ganglia. Although these brain areas are

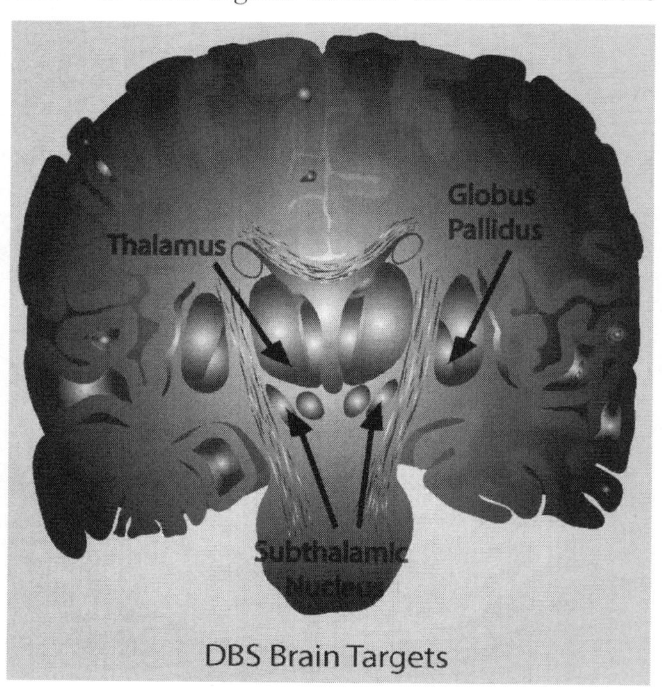

DBS Brain Targets

interrelated, target selection differs depending on the person's symptoms and medication complexity. For instance, when stimulating the Vim, tremor is greatly diminished or stopped. The STN and GPi are brain areas commonly selected in PD since stimulation can reduce stiffness (excessive muscle tone), slowness, tremor, and dyskinesia. Stimulation of GPi or STN can improve symptoms of dystonia and related pain or abnormal posturing. Your DBS team will determine which brain area will give the best outcome and result.

When is the right time to consider DBS?

DBS is no longer a *'treatment of last resort.'* In this section we discuss the best time or window of opportunity for DBS to improve symptoms and quality of life. If DBS is performed after this time when symptoms have reached a severe stage, the chance for optimal benefit may have passed. There is no specific age limit for surgery but factors such as general health, symptom severity, cognitive (thinking) function and other medical problems must be considered when determining the safety of surgery.

The decision to have surgery includes more than just an analysis of movement symptoms and severity. Deep brain stimulation can improve symptoms when medicine cannot be increased, and in select cases reduce reliance on medications and related side effects. The burden of medication used to treat tremor, PD or dystonia can also be costly and cause serious side effects that limit how much medication can be taken. Medications can cause nausea, dizziness, leg swelling, sedation, fatigue, confusion, hallucinations and impulse control problems. A consultation with a medical team that specializes in DBS will help determine your risks and benefits.

Jill's Advice

"Having Parkinson's disease is not a choice but you do have treatment choices. One such option is Deep Brain Stimulation (DBS). If you are considering DBS, you are on the precipice of a decision that may dramatically change your life for the better. However, having made the decision to have this surgery myself, I know first-hand how frightening the road ahead can be. Positive DBS success rates and study results are all well and good, but making that leap to voluntarily have a hole drilled in your head, when you are more or less doing well, may not be the obvious choice. Let me tell you how sure I am that having DBS was the right

decision for me.

I was you. Doing all the right things; exercising, eating right, trying all sorts of alternative treatments and functioning pretty well. Or so I thought. I told myself that I could live with the limitations Parkinson's disease threw at me. But after eight years, my symptoms were clearly getting worse and my medications were simultaneously increasing and becoming less effective. I had finally had enough…

Enough to do the extreme and say yes to DBS. And am I glad I did. And so is everyone else in my life, including my husband, my kids, my friends and my colleagues at work. So ask yourself these questions:

Are you truly okay living this compromised life? Are you tired of not sleeping through the night because of movement problems or frequent medication dosing? Are you tired of your tremor intensifying at the worst of times? Do you want to be social again and enjoy the activities you've given up?

For me, having DBS was like getting glasses, "Oh, this is how normal people see!" I had actually forgotten what it felt like not to be in some level of pain. Can I tell you what a joy it is to finally feel good and like I have been given my life back? I am so thrilled with the results that I would literally be willing to have the surgery again every month just to feel this way.

Is it scary? Of course it is… it is a very serious surgery and without a doubt the most frightening thing I have ever done in my life. And although you are getting a hole drilled into your head, it actually is not all that risky. With a fatality rate of up to 1.3%, you are actually more likely to die in a car accident or from heart disease than have major complications due to DBS. Still, no matter how it is rationalized, this is a serious surgery.

Everyone I have spoken to who has had DBS has told me it was the best decision they ever made and that they only wish they hadn't waited so long. Add me to that list of proponents.

So stop waiting, get the facts, learn if DBS is for you and take the steps to get your life back. I'm so glad I did."
-Jill Ater

Parkinson's and DBS

Parkinson's disease (PD) is caused by dopamine nerve cell loss in the basal ganglia. Problems such as tremor, muscle rigidity (stiffness and spasms) and slowness of movement appear as dopamine levels decline over time. The role of DBS in Parkinson's disease can be best understood through a discussion of three stages of disability, *mild*, *moderate* and *advanced.* Understanding these stages and how they apply to your situation can help you stratify the risk versus benefit when considering DBS surgery.

MILD-STAGE. In the mild or early stage, levodopa or dopamine enhancing medications effectively improve motor symptoms throughout the day. Movements are often controlled with little to no variability (variability is called fluctuations) in response to each dose. In fact, many people do not notice that their next dose is due and must make special efforts to take medication on schedule. Of course people with Parkinson's can still have 'good' and 'bad' days or find that their symptoms change in situations associated with stress, fatigue or illness. DBS is not usually recommended at this stage since medicine is effective and the risk of brain surgery outweighs the potential benefit. Sometimes tremor can be difficult to treat even when medication improves other movement symptoms. Deep brain stimulation is sometimes considered earlier if tremor is disabling despite adequate medication and control of other symptoms. If DBS were to slow some aspects of progression, then perhaps the benefit would outweigh the risk of having brain surgery but this is not proven. Considering DBS during mild stages of PD, comes down to risk. The most important question at this stage – *Are my symptoms bad enough or bothersome enough to justify the risks of brain surgery?*

Practical Tips: Think about how you move and what you cannot do when you take your medications. Does each dose improve your symptoms as expected or are you under-medicated? Are you experiencing medication side effects that are limiting the amount of medication you can tolerate? Deep brain stimulation may be considered sooner if you are experiencing intolerable medication side effects.

MODERATE-STAGE. Deep brain stimulation is most helpful in the moderate stage. In this stage, medication doses continue to improve symptoms such as tremor, rigidity, slow movement, shuffling and posture. However, the time that each medication dose is effective becomes shorter;

often not lasting from one dose to the next, an effect referred to as *end of dose wearing off*. When the benefits of medication wear off between doses the medication must be increased or taken more often. Dyskinesia can occur as medications are increased. Dyskinesia are involuntary (unintentional) or jerky motions caused by dopamine medication. Dyskinesia typically occurs when medication levels (levodopa) are at their peak, but can also occur when medications levels are wearing off. Like dyskinesia, dystonia (abrupt muscle spasm, contraction or twisting) can occur at peak dose or when the dose is wearing off.

Deep brain stimulation surgery is best considered when medications still work yet the effect wears off before the next dose or dyskinesia limits further doses. Stimulation improves the same symptoms that improve with medication. An important point to remember is that symptoms that do not improve with dopaminergic medication (levodopa) do not typically improve with stimulation. In other words, DBS is as *good as medication* but the effect of stimulation does not wear off like medications. The difference between stimulation and medication is that stimulation allows for smoother control of symptoms, less reliance on medication, less medication side effects, less dyskinesia, less tremor and less medication costs.

Practical Tips: ***Think about how you move and what you can do when your medications are working. This is how DBS can impact your daily life. If your medications do not help your balance, freezing of gait, speech or falling, DBS will not help these symptoms either and surgery could even make them worse. Tremor and dystonia are exceptions in that these symptoms may not respond to medicine but do respond to DBS.***

ADVANCED-STAGE. Over time, some of the most bothersome and disabling symptoms become less responsive to dopaminergic medications. At this stage, advanced symptoms such as falling, poor balance, gait freezing, speech and swallowing problems typically do not improve with more medication and do not improve with stimulation. Understanding which of your symptoms still improve with medication is critical to understanding which symptoms will improve with stimulation.

This is very important as growing disability prompts many people to seek out DBS due to frustration at this stage and this frustration increases one's desperation to '*try-anything*'. Understanding the limitations of DBS is also important if you already have DBS and are expecting DBS to help symptoms of advanced stage or disease progression. You may hope or want

DBS to improve advanced symptoms when medications are not helpful. Rehabilitation therapy can be very helpful when symptoms refractory to medication and surgery such as imbalance, freezing of gait, speech or swallowing problems increase. You can learn more about these therapies in chapter 7.

Practical Tips: Deep brain stimulation should not be considered as a treatment of last resort as the benefit is less; the risk of brain surgery is greater in advanced disease and can result in worsening balance, gait, falling, cognition and speech problems.

The following exercise will explore your symptoms and expectations for DBS. If you already have DBS, this exercise will help you determine if you are getting optimal benefit or expecting too much from DBS. Any symptom that improves with medication should also improve with stimulation.

SYMPTOMS & EXPECTATIONS EXERCISE

The first step is to list the top 3 symptoms or expectations (symptoms or activities) that you, your care-partner and Neurologist want from DBS therapy.

My expectations for improvement with DBS

1.
2.
3.

My care-partner's or family's expectations for improvement with DBS

1.
2.
3.

My Neurologist's expectations for improvement with DBS

1.
2.
3.

Put an 'X' in the column that corresponds to the symptom you would like DBS to improve and whether the symptom improves with medications.

Parkinson's Symptom	Is a symptom I want DBS to improve	Improves with dopamine medication	Does not improve with dopamine medication	Neurologist comment section: symptoms that should improve
Stiff Muscles				
Slow Movement				
Tremor		Should improve		
Muscle Cramps				
Pain				
Shuffling				
Speech				
Swallowing				
Gait Freezing				
Imbalance				
Falling				
Cognition				
Depression				
Anxiety				
Insomnia				
Dyskinesia		Should improve		

The above exercises allow a general assessment of the symptoms that are expected to respond to DBS and your expectations for improvement with DBS. Symptoms that improve with medication also typically improve with stimulation. Be sure to compare your expectations and that of your care-partner and Neurologist's to insure DBS can meet your expectations. (Note: This exercise can also be helpful many years after DBS when evaluating symptoms of disease progression.) Your answers will guide your treatment discussion with your family and your DBS medical team.

Medication Reduction

Medication reduction may be one of your goals for surgery. Medication reduction is possible especially with STN stimulation. The elimination of all PD medications is not common and in some cases can be harmful since under-dosing medication places a higher demand on the brain and body to manage without dopamine. In general, medicine reduction is greater in people with milder symptoms or when tremor is the predominating symptom.

Discussion Topics for Parkinson's Disease

Understanding the limits of DBS is very important before surgery and with disease progression.

Parkinson's symptoms that do not respond well to PD medication typically do not respond to DBS. Tremor is an exception since tremor responds well to stimulation.

Optimal benefit may take up to 6 or 9 months depending on individual symptoms.

Balance, posture, speech, swallowing and walking problems occur in advancing PD. DBS is not typically helpful for these symptoms of progression and rehabilitation therapy is even more important in your care.

DBS is not considered a treatment for non-motor symptoms such as depression, thinking problems, hallucinations, bladder problems, constipation or fatigue.

Rarely, surgery can worsen walking and/or balance. This is not possible to predict prior to DBS surgery.

Death is a rare complication of DBS surgery.

Tremor

Tremors are unintentional rhythmic movements in one or more parts of your body. Tremor is usually seen in the hands but can also occur in the arm, leg, foot, body, head, face, and vocal cords (voice.) Hand tremor is further differentiated by whether it occurs when your arm/hand is at rest (seen in Parkinson's disease) or when you are actively using your hands for tasks (seen with Essential tremor or some forms of secondary tremor). Tremor can occur at any age but is most common in middle-aged and older people. Initially tremor can be mild and be dismissed as a problem of fatigue, over-exertion, anxiety or stress.

Some families have tremor that is noted over many generations and some people with tremor have no known cause. Genetic or inherited forms of tremor respond well to DBS. Secondary tremor is less responsive to DBS. Examples of secondary tremor include tremor associated with medical conditions such as an overactive thyroid, liver disease, head injury, stroke, multiple sclerosis, heavy metal poisoning, vitamin deficiency and certain medications. Although some people find that alcohol improves tremor, excessive or long-term alcohol use can eventually worsen tremor and cause other health and cognitive problems.

Tremor is not a life threatening condition but can be very disabling and isolating. The simplest yet most important part of your daily routine can become impossible, such as getting dressed, eating, drinking, writing or reading. For some, the use of medications to reduce tremor can interact with other medications or are limited by side effects such as sedation, dizziness, imbalance and confusion.

DBS is appropriate when medications are not effective enough to reduce tremor or when medication side effects are intolerable. Thalamic stimulation can improve your ability to do routine daily tasks, reduce social isolation and minimize medicine side effects. Tremor characteristics vary and some forms of tremor respond better to stimulation than others. An experienced DBS team can review whether your tremor characteristics will respond well to DBS.

Discussion Topics for Tremor

Thalamic (VIM) DBS is a treatment for tremor.

Tremor improves quickly with just a few stimulation adjustments.

DBS may not stop tremor completely.

Benefit from DBS depends on the characteristic and location of the tremor.

DBS does not improve balance.

DBS can work even if medications do not help and most people can greatly reduce or gradually stop tremor medications after DBS.

A clear understanding about what tasks DBS can improve and how DBS will impact your symptoms over time is very important before having surgery.

DBS can cause speech or balance problems. This is not possible to predict prior to DBS surgery although these problems are most commonly caused by inappropriate stimulation.

Death is a rare complication of DBS surgery.

Dystonia

Dystonia is a complex and chronic condition that affects muscles and joints. Dystonia is a term used to describe a sustained involuntary muscle contraction or spasm that can cause twisting, bending or flexion of your joint(s). The muscles cannot relax normally and contractions can cause abnormal postures of the arms, legs, hands, feet neck and body. This results in pain, limited or abnormal movement.

Dystonia can involve the whole body (generalized) or just part of the body (focal.) An example of focal dystonia is cervical dystonia otherwise called torticollis. Cervical dystonia affects the neck and head position sparing other areas of the body. Dystonia can also be brought on by specific activities or tasks such as hand dystonia experienced while writing or playing a musical instrument. This is called task specific dystonia.

Dystonia can be a primary problem or can be a symptom associated with a medical condition such as stroke, Multiple Sclerosis or Parkinson's. Dystonia occurs in men and women equally and can begin at any age.

There is no cure for dystonia. Medications can help; however, medications can be limited by side effects. Many clinicians recommend a trial of medication or botulinum toxin (i.e., Botox®, Myobloc®) before DBS surgery.

Dystonia has many causes and different types of dystonia will respond differently to DBS. Factors associated with surgical success include whether dystonia is a primary condition (often genetic), secondary to another condition, time of onset, degree of pain and location of dystonia. In general primary dystonia responds best to DBS. Dyskinesia and dystonia secondary to medications sometimes referred to as tardive dyskinesia or dystonia can also respond to DBS. Because dystonia can be difficult to diagnosis and in some cases DBS outcomes are difficult to predict, the evaluation process and long-term DBS care should be conducted by a medical team that is highly experienced in both DBS and dystonia. Dystonia improves more slowly with stimulation often taking 6 to 12 months to improve.

Discussion Topics for Dystonia

DBS is a beneficial treatment for primary dystonia (inherited forms of dystonia usually respond very well to DBS).

Secondary forms of dystonia (caused by another condition) do not generally respond as well to DBS. The exception is medication induced tardive dyskinesia or dystonia may respond to DBS.

DBS is not a cure for dystonia.

Dystonia improves slowly once stimulation is set and can take up to 12 months to see full benefit.

DBS can work even if dystonia medications do not help and many people can reduce or stop their dystonia medications after DBS.

A clear understanding about what DBS can improve is very important before having brain surgery.

Surgery can cause walking and/or balance problems. This is not possible to predict prior to DBS surgery.

Death is a rare complication of DBS surgery.

Alice's Encouragement

Sing as if no one is listening, love like you've never been hurt, dance like no one is watching, and live everyday as if it were your last!

"That's stitched on an old sampler hanging in my kitchen and every morning I read it and think how lucky I am that I have PD. I was diagnosed December 1998 with Young Onset PD disease and if I had known then what I know now I think I would have handled things a bit different. My DBS units were implanted December 2007; they changed my life and gave me more years to be me, funny term huh – to be me. This disease changes you, and your family; some good some bad but always a rollercoaster ride. The sooner the better for DBS I think.

'Never say Never' – not me no one is going to drill a hole in my head let alone two!! I have only thrown myself out of bed once since the DBS implants. I'm not in a wheelchair now and I'm driving in the daytime, quilting, watercolor painting and making my cards. Here's hoping that you and your families understand that this is a slow journey with many turns and bumps in the road. You feel something then stop and get a look at the bump, thinking hey that doesn't look so big, I can handle it and you do, then next you hit another head on- not the smartest thing to do, but you managed and then another and then you decided to slow down some, cause the bumps seem to become bigger or closer together…You're thinking "Why me?"

You and your family can learn as little or as much as you want – it's out there for you to sponge it up – knowledge is power. So I say learn all you can and keep the hope; remember this affects the entire family, not just you but those you love and love you… I finally learned that I am not the same person – how could I be? I do what I can when I can and the rest will have to wait…some days I can make lemonade, and other days I don't have the ice or sugar and am too shaky for adding the water…take care, hugs to you all."

-Alice Cleeton

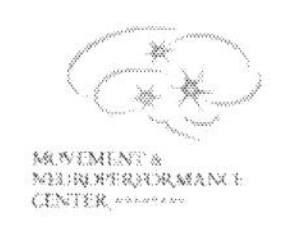

NOTES

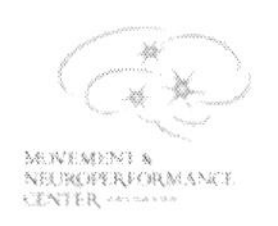

2 THE SURGERY EVALUATION

"I was diagnosed with early onset Parkinson's in 1996. I managed my symptoms through medication, exercise and a positive attitude. Eventual I felt like my medications were causing more problems than they were solving. I was constantly dyskinetic, it was difficult to do simple tasks or even hold a decent conversation. I underwent DBS surgery in 2008. Now (4) years later, I can honestly say "This was the best decision I, my wife and our four children ever made."

-Michael Erb

This section will guide you through a typical DBS surgery evaluation, describe the DBS medical team, their role in the evaluation and the rationale behind tests and procedures that are performed as you and your team considers whether surgery is right for you. Although the DBS evaluation will differ between centers, most clinics use a team approach to provide collective expertise and opinion as to whether DBS is the right next step in your treatment. The following specialists and procedures are an important part of the pre-surgical DBS evaluation.

Practical Tips: Be prepared. Bring someone with you to take notes. Bring copies of exercises you completed in chapter one. Ask any questions that remain unanswered. Examples of questions to ask during your evaluation are at the end of this chapter.

Neurology Consult: A neurologist specialized in movement disorders and DBS is usually the first team member you will see for consultation. The neurologist will complete the following:

- Confirm your diagnosis
- Assess whether adequate medical treatments have been tried
- Measure the severity of your symptoms
- Identify the symptoms DBS can improve
- Discuss your expectations for DBS
- Explain the process of adjusting the stimulation over time

- Review the neurostimulator battery options
- Review general risks for brain surgery
- Review expected benefits and alternative treatment options
- Refer to other healthcare professionals as indicated

Off-On Levodopa Medication Testing *(Parkinson's disease only):* If you have PD, a special appointment is needed to evaluate and compare your symptoms when medications are very low and when medications are peaking in your body. This appointment is typically scheduled early in the morning so the examination can occur before you take your first medication dose of the day. Your symptoms are evaluated and given a severity score. You then take your morning dose of PD medications and another examination and score is noted once this dose has taken effect. This evaluation documents the severity of your symptoms off and on medication to help define more clearly the symptoms that improve with medication (as we have reviewed in the prior chapter, these are the same symptoms predicted to improve with DBS). The most important symptoms that are assessed during this appointment include walking, balance, stiffness, tremor, dyskinesia, speech, posture, muscle spasms, mood and blood pressure. Medication side effects are also noted.

Practical Tips: ***When you arrive for your Off-On testing appointment, make sure you notify your clinician if your medications have not completely worn off. You may need to extend the observation time before you take your morning dose of medication. Do not hold or delay medications you take for other serious medical conditions (such as blood pressure or diabetes) unless specifically informed to hold all medications by your neurologist. The outcome of this evaluation identifies which symptoms will or will not improve with surgery. Ask you medical team to review their findings and conclusions from this test with you.***

Significance for you: The Off-On evaluation gives you and your neurologist the opportunity to discuss your expectations for DBS. The symptoms that improve when you take your PD medications should also improve with stimulation (with the exception of tremor since DBS can help tremor even when medicines do not). The evaluation also establishes a baseline or time point that can be useful for comparison to determine if you have reached your optimal benefit with stimulation the first year after surgery.

Practical Tips: If you are experiencing problems after DBS, an off-on medication evaluation can help you and your doctor understand if stimulation is optimal, determine if you are taking adequate medication dosages and whether disease progression is the underlying problem.

Significance for your neurologist and neurosurgeon: Your neurologist will observe the severity of your symptoms without medication and improvement experienced after your medication dose. This observation provides the following helpful information:

- An improvement in symptoms after taking medication helps confirm your diagnosis of PD.
- Identify symptoms DBS will help based on response to medication.
- Determine the brain target that would be the best for you.
- Determine if surgery is required on one or both sides.

The following example describes how this information can be used. If you are living with DBS and begin to experience problems with balance or gait freezing, the question arises: do you need more medication, more intense stimulation, is the disease progressing or are you experiencing a stimulation side effect? Off-on medicine testing helps answer these questions even years after DBS. This knowledge about your symptoms will help avoid the tendency to adjust stimulation frequently for symptoms that will not improve and avoid unnecessary side effects and frustration for you and your neurologist.

Practical Tips: Complete the Symptoms & Expectations Worksheet found in the prior chapter and bring to your neurology or programming appointments. Ask your neurologist or programmer to complete their section and discuss the results. Review these results with your care-partner or family so they too can understand the role of DBS in your life.

Neuropsychological Evaluation: Neuropsychological testing measures your thinking (cognitive) abilities. Significant thinking problems can increase your risk of confusion during or after surgery. A neuropsychologist will aid your team in determining this risk.

The neuropsychologist will also ask about particular emotional symptoms that may increase the complexity of your care after DBS such as impulse control problems, hallucinations, delusions, anxiety, depression, suicide thoughts or attempts, panic attacks and mania. Your mood must be stable before DBS surgery. Untreated or unstable hallucinations, delusions, depression and/or anxiety can significantly increase your risk during surgery and after surgery when stimulation is adjusted. A psychiatrist or counselor may be required before surgery depending on your symptoms.

Significance for you: DBS is an elective surgery. Gathering as much information as possible before surgery helps mitigate risk, allows you time to make an informed decision about whether DBS is the right choice for you or seek additional treatment. Untreated anxiety can lead to panic attacks at time of surgery. Untreated depression may leave you feeling poorly even if DBS improves your movement symptoms. Cognitive problems can worsen during or after surgery. DBS may not be recommended if dementia is diagnosed during your evaluation, although there are exceptions depending on the severity of dementia and other medical factors.

Significance for your neurologist and neurosurgeon: The neuropsychological evaluation measures your baseline thinking abilities and emotional wellbeing prior to surgery. There are instances when cognitive weaknesses or emotional instability increase surgical risk beyond what is acceptable. When risk outweighs the potential benefit, the probability to cause harm is high and DBS is not recommended.

Video Exam: A video record of your baseline examination is sometimes performed to document the severity of your symptoms prior to DBS and provides a video for comparison when monitoring improvement after DBS. This can be especially helpful for complex symptoms such as dystonia and tremor.

DBS Counseling: A DBS counseling appointment is strongly recommended before surgery. This wrap-up appointment gives you the opportunity to ask any remaining questions, discuss what to expect before, during and after surgery, review risks, benefits, review your general health and the long-term care and stimulation appointments after DBS. During the counseling appointment you can also learn about DBS neurostimulator options, occupational, environmental and medical safety guidelines. The counseling appointment can be conducted by your neurologist, neurosurgeon, nurse or physician assistant involved in your care.

Practical Tips: Ask for another appointment if you are not clear about the surgery, risks and programming schedule after surgery.

Brain Imaging: A brain MRI will be performed if not recently done. If brain MRI is contraindicated due to other implanted devices (heart pacemaker), a head CT scan will be performed. Brain imaging is used to assess for any structural anomalies or prior brain damage that may limit the safety of DBS surgery.

Neurosurgery Consult: A neurosurgeon specialized in DBS surgery will review your evaluation data and provide you with another opinion about how DBS surgery will impact your symptoms. The neurosurgeon will also discuss the following:

- Explain the details of the procedure
- Review your brain MRI or head CT scan
- Review how many procedures s/he has done and their outcomes
- General risk and complication rates
- His or her personal experience with complications
- His or her personal experience and preference of brain targets
- Expected post-operative care

The neurosurgeon will explain the sequence of events the day of the surgery and the surgical technique that will be used to implant the wire. S/he will discuss who will be in the operating room and about how long the procedure may take. The surgical team will work with your insurance payer to obtain authorization for the surgery.

General Health Screening: A general health screen by your primary care physician should be completed prior to scheduling your DBS surgery to avoid last minute surgery cancellations or delays. Lab tests, chest X-ray, EKG or stress test may be needed depending on your age and general health. This is also an opportunity for you to ask your primary care whether there is any cause to obtain a body MRI as this currently cannot be obtained after DBS. (Note: researchers are studying the safety of body MRI after DBS so this may change in the future.)

Dental Check-up: The authors also recommend a dental check-up if not done in the prior year or if you are experiencing problems with tooth pain, decay or have fractured teeth. Dental work completed before surgery improves your overall health, nutrition and reduces the risk of infection if a dental abscess or dental procedure occurs shortly after DBS surgery.

Precautions: At the time of our manuscript, body MRI cannot be performed after DBS due to risk of brain damage or death. Inform your primary care doctor or specialist about this restriction and review any potential needs you may have for MRI imaging. For example, an MRI could be helpful to determine the cause of ongoing joint, neck or back pain so it would be important to discuss whether an MRI is needed prior to DBS.

Health History: Make a list of your allergies, prescribed medications, all vitamins, home remedies, supplements and over-the-counter medications for your neurologist and bring to the hospital on the morning of surgery. Inform your medical team of any personal history or family history of seizures, prior brain surgery, stroke, heart attack, heart stent, heart valve problems or heart surgery, implanted hardware, blood clots, high blood pressure, hepatitis, excessive bleeding or bruising, fainting, blood transfusion, skin or other infection or past problems with anesthesia. Report if anyone in your family has a bleeding disorder. Be sure to inform your team of prior history or ongoing problem with hallucinations, depressed mood, panic attacks or suicidal thoughts before DBS surgery.

Practical Tips: Inform your medical team if you are taking aspirin or other medications to keep blood from clotting. Your team will tell you when to stop and restart these medications after surgery. Be sure to include supplements and over the counter medicines on your medication list as some may increase bleeding risk (i.e. gingko biloba, Pepto bismol, St. Johns Wort, and garlic are a few examples).

TIMELINE DEPICTING TYPICAL DBS EVALUATION

-1 to -6 Months	*Neurology Consultation* *Off-On Evaluation (PD Only)* *Rehabilitation (if indicated)* *Neuropsychology Evaluation* *Primary Care Check Up & Dental Check Up* *Brain MRI* *Neurosurgical Consultation* *Special Clearances (i.e. Cardiology)* *Labs and exam for hospitalization* *Pre-Admission hospital appointment*
Day 0	*Brain Surgery – Lead Implantation*
Day 1-3	*Hospital Stay*
Day 7-21	*Suture Removal and neurostimulator battery implantation (out-patient surgery)*
Day 21-30	*Healing Phase - First programming adjustment typically occurs after the 'honeymoon' or microlesion effect has subsided, skin still under close monitoring*
Month 2-12	*Optimization Phase (adjustments every 2-4 weeks until optimal settings reached), rehabilitation, medication adjustments, exercise, education, optimize health status*
Month >12	*Maintenance Phase – Battery and hardware checks, skin checks, rehabilitation maintenance*

Be prepared: Ask Questions Before DBS

Questions to ask your DBS Neurologist

1. Am I a fair, good or excellent candidate?
2. What is involved in the evaluation?
3. Who is on the team?
4. When is the right time for DBS?
5. What are the alternatives to DBS?
6. Will I be able to reduce my medications and how much?
7. What will improve after surgery and how long will it take?
8. How many appointments will it take to finish the adjustments?
9. What is your experience with surgical complications and rates?
10. Will DBS limit my opportunities to participate in research?
11. Who are the top surgeons in my area with great results?
12. Which of my symptoms are not at all likely to improve?
13. What is your preferred neurostimulator battery and why?
14. Do you prefer I have one or both sides of my brain implanted?
15. How many patients do you have with DBS?
16. Who will be adjusting my stimulation settings?
17. When should my neurostimulator be turned on after surgery?
18. Do you have a preference of surgical technique?
19. What brain target will help my symptoms the most and why?
20. Will you see me in the hospital if I have a surgical complication?

Questions to ask your programmer

1. How long do you like to wait to turn on the stimulation?
2. How long will the programming appointments last?
3. Is DBS the focus of your practice?
4. Who supervises if you are not an MD, PA or NP?
5. How many patients have you programmed?
6. How many different brain targets have you programmed?
7. Which of my symptoms will improve with stimulation?
8. How many sessions does it take to reach optimal settings?
9. Where did you receive your training to adjust the stimulation?
10. What do you do if the stimulation doesn't work as expected?
11. Do you have any concerns about my risk during surgery?
12. What do you do if stimulation doesn’t work out for me?
13. Who can see me if you are not available?
14. If I have a problem, how long does it take to see you?
15. Who do I call if I have a questions or problem with stimulation?

Questions to ask your DBS Neurosurgeon

1. Who is on your team and who will be in the operating room?
2. How long until the surgery can be scheduled?
3. How many trips will I have to make to your office or hospital?
4. What are the steps involved in the surgical process?
5. How long does your typical surgery last?
6. How many **people** have you implanted with STN, GPi or Vim?
7. What are your complication percentages?
8. Have any of your patients died within a few days of having DBS?
9. What percentage of improvement is average for your patients?
10. Who do I call if I have problems after surgery?
11. How many of your patients required repositioning of the wire?
12. How long have you been doing DBS surgery?
13. Where did you receive your training to do DBS surgery?
14. Who do you recommend to adjust the stimulation after surgery?
15. Which surgeon do you recommend if I want a second opinion?
16. How much time during the surgery will I be asleep or awake?
17. Will you use MRI or CT, frame or frameless technique?
18. When is the neurostimulator implanted?
19. How long has your preferred surgical technique been approved, tested, researched or proven to be the most effective technique in assuring that I will have the best possible outcome?

Questions to ask yourself

1. What do I really want to make better with DBS?
2. Which of my symptoms respond to my PD medications?
3. Will improving these symptoms justify the risk of surgery?
4. Can I make it to the required programming appointments?
5. Does my lifestyle allow for living with implanted hardware?
6. How many patients have I talked to that have DBS?
7. Were they happy with their decision to have DBS?
8. Is my family supportive with my decision to have DBS?
9. Do I have mood problems that may increase my risks?
10. Do I have any hallucinations that I haven't told my doctor?
11. Can I deal with a significant improvement in my symptoms?
12. I have had opportunity to ask all my questions about DBS?
13. I feel absolutely confident I am making the right decision?
14. I have chosen the right DBS team for me?
15. I understand my walking, balance or thinking could get worse?
16. I could have a serious complications and I have discussed this with my doctor?

Gayle's Story
Living with the Mehren's Shakes

"When I was growing up I remember my mother, most of her siblings, and her father with tremors in their hands, head, and voice. When I asked about them I was always told they were the 'Mehren's shakes'. My Mother's maiden name was Mehrens. In 1998 (shortly after my 50th birthday) I noticed the tremors in my hands and I thought okay so I have the family Mehren's shakes.

In 2007 my tremors were getting worse so I decided to see a Neurologist. She told me my "Mehren's Shakes" were really familial essential tremors. Familial because I inherited them from my family. I don't know why they call them essential because I could live my life very nicely without them. But tremors they are! I was informed there are no drugs for tremors so doctors " borrow" medicines from other conditions such as Parkinson's. The neurologist ordered a sleep deprivation study and a brain MRI. Those tests showed nothing irregular. I was put on a drug called clonazepam, told to try that for a couple of months and return to see how the medication helped.

Armed with a real name for my condition I turned to the internet to see what I could find. The first thing I found was an organization called International Essential (there's that word again!) Tremor Foundation better known as IETF. I joined that organization and began receiving information about what other people were doing to cope and tips on how to "live" with this condition. Another tidbit I read about was a procedure called Deep Brain Stimulation or DBS. I vowed I would not let anyone probe around in my brain. That was just too radical. I returned to my Neurologist and told her that the drug was not working; I was not seeing any change except in my motivation. I seemed to be tired a lot more. She prescribed Propranolol and said to return in 2 months. There still was no change except I was even more tired. Once again I was put on a third drug, primidone, and told to return in 2 months. This went on for about a year just increasing the dosage of these meds. The tremors continued to increase.

By late 2010 I told my Neurologist that we needed to do something different, the current meds were not working and side effects were becoming a problem. I was beginning to have head and voice tremors. She said she had done all she could and sent me to a university center for a second opinion. They felt she was on the right track and that I should increase my primidone from 300 mg to 1000 mg a day. Side effects were becoming a problem. My balance and cognition was impacted by all the meds. Meantime, I could no longer write my name. I quit my job as I could no longer type on a computer or dial a phone. I could no longer play the piano. Eating became a "sharing of everything on my plate." I would tell my fellow diners that I hope their "ducking" skills were good as I would surely share!

My next ray of hope came in the fall of 2012. I received notice of a new support group for tremor. I attended the meeting and was excited about what the team had to offer and the care and concern they have. I had the opportunity to talk with a gentleman who had DBS surgery and was impressed with what he had to say. The next day after discussing the options with my husband we decided to make an appointment with Dr. Giroux and see what she had to say. We met with Dr. Giroux and Sierra Farris. Dr. Giroux was very concerned about side effects and we had a serious conversation about the number of and high doses of medicines. She had both my and Dale's attention. While she didn't make any recommendations, she did tell us what options were available and DBS was one of them.

With this information, we went home and discussed DBS with our primary care physician advised us to interview Neurosurgeons, Neurologists and the teams that would work with me after the surgery. And the interviewing began. My first step was to define my expectations from the surgery and find out what was realistic and what probably would not happen. I created an Excel spread sheet with a list of my activities and columns for yes, no, and maybe.

I gathered "props" and took them to my next appointment. I am a fly fisherman and I can't tie my own fly on my leader, so I took a fly and my leader. I do ceramics and could no longer paint my projects to finish them, so I took a ceramic piece. I play competitive bridge and could no longer hold 13 cards and I took a deck of cards. I didn't need to take a pen and paper as they could see I could not write. Now armed with my spreadsheet and props, my husband and I started "interviewing" Neurosurgeons and Neurologists.

During my DBS evaluation, I was told that I needed to change the "yes" column heading to "maybe yes". The team cautioned me that DBS would be more successful treating hand tremor than my head or voice tremors as they are "core" tremors. Also along the way I found a book "Living with a Battery Operated Brain" written by a patient with Parkinson's and her story. While she had Parkinson's and I have Essential Tremor, I found a lot of useful and information in the book. Armed with information and realistic expectations, I was ready to take the next step.

IT TIME. LET'S DO THIS THING!!!

I arrived at the hospital at 5:00 a.m. for my 7:30a.m. surgery and was immediately met by a team of doctors, nurses, and the anesthesiologist. My halo was placed on my head and I was taken to get an MRI then off to the O.R. While I needed to be awake for most of the surgery, I was never in any pain or uncomfortable. Being awake made me feel like I was part of the "fix". I had some important input to finding the "sweet spot". ..

Sierra asked me to do the lovely spiral that always looked like a flowering rose and after stimulation actually looked like a spiral! Next was the strait line. It actually looked like a line and not waves on the ocean. Then came "write your name". I could write my name and it was readable! I started to cry. I woke up in the recovery room and the nurse asked me if I wanted some ice chips. When she handed me a glass of ice, I looked at her and thought "this won't work". I looked around to see who I was going to "share" my ice chips with and luckily it was just me. But my fears quickly washed away as I fed myself those ice chips, WITH A SPOON!!! It was a beautiful thing!

I have been living with DBS now for almost a year. My head, hand and voice tremor is negligible. I have my quality of life back. It was nothing short of a miracle in my book! I am blessed and oh so thankful! I am back to doing my fused glass artistry, fly fishing, playing duplicate bridge, sewing (as I can once again thread my sewing machine), drinking with one hand, and yes- writing my name. I think it is important to mention that I have no speech or gait problems; actually my balance is better now that I am off the tremor medicines. My recommendations for anyone considering DBS:

- *Do your homework. Learn about the surgery and what it can do for you. This book is a good first step.*
- *Assemble your team. Interview neurologists, neurosurgeons, programmers. Find a comprehensive team that you feel comfortable with and that you can talk to and that listens; a team that treats the whole person, not just a DBS patient. You will have a long bond with this group.*
- *Set your goals. What do you really want to do that you can't do now? Press your Neurosurgeon and Neurologist for a realistic answer. Don't have surgery with undefined or unvoiced expectations.*
- *Talk to DBS patients; attend support groups to see what others have to say.*
- *And most importantly, go in with a positive attitude."*

-Gayle Schendzielos

NOTES

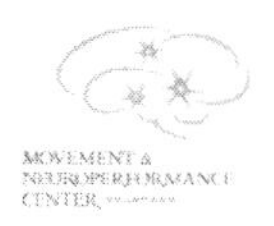

3 THE SURGERY

How bad is "bad enough" to undergo DBS?

This is a common question asked by people considering DBS surgery and people that have been denied DBS because they were told *"you are not bad enough."* So how bad is bad enough to undergo DBS surgery? The answer is complex and requires a review of diagnosis, symptom severity, optimal use of medication and other therapy, potential benefits, long-term care access, personal expectations, fears, readiness and risks. If surgery is not offered because symptoms are "too mild" consider making a list of activities you have difficulty performing, medication side affects you are dealing with and the total time you feel pain or off time for your doctor. A second opinion is always an option if you feel the time is right for DBS.

What are the surgical risks?

The following risks are the most common and can be used to guide your discussion of risk with your surgeon. This list is not complete so be sure to learn about your surgeon's experience with risks, their frequency of complications and other risks that would be unique to your situation. The rate of complications in this section is taken from high volume DBS centers that report their experiences with surgical complications.

Hemorrhage. Bleeding in the brain is one of the most serious complications. The risk of hemorrhage reported in research publications ranges from 1 to 2% with less than 1% on average leading to permanent problems. This percentage should not be applied to all surgeons and all hospitals that offer DBS. Ask your surgeon for his/her specific rate of hemorrhage and how many total lead wire implants they have performed.

Infection: Infection rates will vary between surgeons and from one hospital to another. Infection rates reported in the literature range from 0% to greater than 15%. Infection can occur superficially on the skin requiring only a short course of oral antibiotics or can be very serious requiring intravenous antibiotics and removal of the DBS hardware. Infections that lead to hardware removal and prolonged antibiotics are the most serious of infections and a comparison of surgeon's rate of infection will help you determine where to have DBS surgery. Each DBS center should give you accurate information about their specific type and rate of DBS post-operative infections and DBS system removals.

Seizure: Seizure occurring during or after DBS surgery is very uncommon and may be associated with bleeding in the brain.

Hardware: Hardware problems include damaged or malfunctioning wires or devices, electrode malposition or migration. The combined risk of hardware complications is about 8% for each brain wire implanted.

Respiratory: Pneumonia, respiratory failure, blood clot or embolism are very uncommon risks that can occur during or after DBS surgery.

Neuropsychiatric: Confusion, delirium, euphoria, depression, mania, personality changes or word finding problems can be temporary or permanent after DBS surgery. Your evaluation prior to DBS can give clues about the risk for these neuropsychiatric complications.

Mobility: New or worsening walking and/or balance problems may be temporary or permanent and is uncommon. Mobility declines after DBS is difficult if not impossible to accurately predict with certainty.

Death: Mortality data is sparse in the community hospital setting. University programs that publish their outcomes consistently report an average risk or death of 0.4%. This is a very rare complication.

Preparing for Surgery - The Waiting Period

This section will guide you through the final steps leading up to surgery and first programming appointment. You will want to confirm that you have insurance coverage for the surgery. Be sure to communicate any changes in your insurance coverage to your surgeon's office. Surgery may be delayed if your health status changes so it is very important to keep your DBS team informed of any changes in your health or medications. *Once you are approved for surgery, it is not uncommon for movement symptoms to be more bothersome as the stress of waiting can be difficult.* Be sure to get plenty of sleep, eat well and limit stress just before surgery.

A Month Or So To Go

See your primary care doctor for a check-up at least one month before surgery. During this appointment you will review your medical issues and treat any problems prior to surgery. At this time, ask whether you have any conditions that might require an MRI since this cannot be done after DBS. An example is an MRI needed to measure arthritis causing joint pain.

Your neurosurgeon's office will provide information about laboratory tests you will need prior to surgery. You will be asked to stop aspirin or other medications that can interfere with blood clotting. It is important that you only stop medications as directed by your surgeon's office.

Practical Tips: Make a complete list of medications, supplements or over-the-counter remedies for review during your consultation for DBS to make sure you are not taking products containing aspirin or blood thinning substances during the time noted by your surgeon.

This is also a good time to make sure your family or home care team is ready. Make plans for time off from work, help with children, cooking, chores, shopping and driving to appointments. You will not be released to drive until all incisions are healed and/or you are considered safe to drive– this may range from 2 to 8 weeks and determined by your surgeon.

Just A Few Days To Go

Try to get as much rest as possible before surgery. You will be asked to take some steps to reduce your risk of infection. For example, you may be asked to use a specific soap or given a body scrub to use in the shower for a few days before surgery to reduce risk of infection. Each surgeon will have a preference for the final preparation before surgery and you should follow his/her directions exactly. *Do not cut or shave your hair unless your surgeon gives you permission.* Ask your surgeon if you should change your medicines the night before or morning of surgery.

Surgery Day Arrives

The day you have been waiting for has arrived. Leave all valuables at home. Do not use any hair or body jells, powders, lotions or creams. If you use a cane, walker or wheelchair, place it in the car for the ride home. When you arrive at the hospital, use a wheelchair if you have any difficulty with your walking or balance. A fall could post-pone your surgery.

After arrival, your anesthesiologist will review your medications, medical history and make sure you have an adequate intravenous line in place to administer fluids and medications during surgery. The next steps will vary and depend on your surgeon's preferences and technique. Surgery is always performed using a targeting or guidance system that may include either a head frame or small pins (fiducials).

Other variables or techniques that may vary depending on your situation and your surgeon's technique include image guided surgery, awake surgery, asleep surgery, unilateral (implantation of one side of the brain) or bilateral (implantation of both side of the brain), single neurostimulator or dual neurostimulators. Surgical techniques are summarized below but your surgeon will review details specific to your planned case.

During surgery, your neurosurgeon will work in the sterile area behind your head. Other members of your DBS team will be by your side in the non-sterile area allowing them to interact with you, examine your symptoms and operate the electrical equipment (if needed). *Report to your surgeon if you experience growing discomfort from your position on the operating table as adjustments in your position can be made during the surgery. Report if you are too warm or too cold or start to experience pain around the pin sites that hold the frame in place, your surgeon can inject more anesthetic into the skin to numb the area to reduce or eliminate any pain.*

Head Frame: Your surgeon will apply anesthetic to your skin and you may receive mild sedation before placing the head frame. Tiny screws (pins) hold the head frame in place. The head frame is required for accuracy in targeting the location to place the electrodes. A brain scan is performed after the head frame is secured to assist with targeting using the frame as a reference. The frame also holds your head steady and allows for some body movement to improve comfort during the procedure. The head frame will be removed immediately after surgery. Additional anesthetic can be given during surgery if the area around the pins becomes uncomfortable.

Frameless: Frameless surgery is an alternative targeting technique. Frameless surgery is a proven method for accurate targeting of the brain regions for DBS. This eliminates the frame that typically obstructs some of your view. The frameless procedure includes the application of navigation markers (fiducial pins) to the skull a day or two before surgery. You will have a brain scan after the fiducials are positioned and you will go home with the fiducials in place. The fiducial pins are used for navigation much like the head frame method and are removed after surgery.

Unilateral vs. Bilateral: When symptoms are bothersome on both sides of the body, you may require stimulation on both sides of the brain for optimal results. Bilateral refers to surgery on both sides of the brain and unilateral refers to surgery on one side. The complications of implanting a side of the brain that is causing little or no symptoms is unknown and the risk to benefit ratio of brain surgery is considerably higher for risk for a less involved side considering there is a risk of permanent damage.

Bilateral Staged or Bilateral Simultaneous: Staged surgery is a term used when only one side of the brain is implanted at a time and when the intention is to ultimately implant both sides. Simultaneous is a term used when both sides of the brain are implanted during one surgery. The decision for staged or simultaneous DBS depends on your symptoms, age, general health, cognitive abilities and surgical risks. Staged surgery reduces the time in the operating room by about a third.

Burr Hole Preparation: A burr hole is required for all DBS surgery techniques to allow for the passage of the DBS wire into the brain. A permanent plastic ring is screwed into the bone. A cap is snapped into the ring which holds the wire in place to prevent the wire from moving and covers the hole to protect the brain. Each wire requires a burr hole. Ask your surgeon if you will be sedated during the preparation of the burr hole. Your surgeon will describe his or her technique with you prior to surgery.

Nerve Cell Recording and Testing: After the burr hole is prepared, you will be awakened for the next step called microelectrode recording (MER). MER is only done for people that undergo awake surgery. MER testing and examination provide valuable information to assist the surgeon in more precisely locating your optimal target to implant the DBS wire by supplementing anatomical information obtained from MRI or CT with your brain's electrical activity or physiologic response. The technical equipment allows the surgeon and neurologist to listen to the electrical signals produced by your neurons and these signals guide the surgeon to the brain target. The neurons produce a sound much like the static of an AM radio. Each brain region has a signature signal which informs the surgeon about the position of the electrode during testing. You will hear these signals amplified using speakers as your team listens to your neurons firing while moving your hand, arm or leg. The photo below is an actual recording strip of an STN neuron during arm movement.

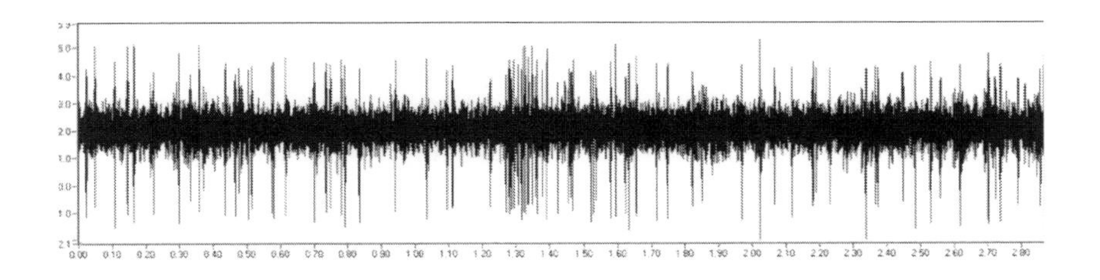

Once nerve cell activity confirms the brain target is reached, stimulation will be turned on to test for beneficial effects and side effects. Testing for side effects is an important step in determining if stimulation will be tolerated later when the stimulation is adjusted in the clinic.

MER allows the surgeon to customize the location of the permanent wire based on your brain anatomy and physiology and informs the surgeon about benefit and undesirable side effects such as speech slurring or thinking changes. If there are undesirable side effects that may limit your benefit, the surgeon may decide to place the wire further away from the area that causes side effects. This part of the procedure may take 30 to 90 minutes. Typical time awake during the actual surgery is usually between 1 to 4 hours. The person is sedated during the remaining time in surgery.

The next step is implantation of the permanent wire into the brain using the information learned from MER. The DBS team will stimulate your brain through the permanent wire while assessing benefit and side effects as a final check insuring accurate placement before finishing the surgery. You will be fully awake for the testing part of the surgery and your symptoms will be assessed frequently. You will be required to provide feedback to the DBS team about how you feel. After stimulation and testing, you will be sedated again for the final closure of the skin.

Image Guided: Image guided implantation is the most recent modification to DBS surgery. Brain MRI or head CT equipment is used to target and implant the electrodes into the brain area while the patient is under anesthesia. Patients remain asleep during the entire procedure and no testing is performed during the implantation of the DBS wire. Image guided technique has become known as *'asleep surgery'* and may provide patients that are uneasy about awake surgery an alternative to being awake. Patients should understand the typical outcomes for DBS have been determined using awake surgery and MER information obtained by testing and examination of the personal individual symptoms.

Unlike MER guided surgery, asleep surgery requires general anesthesia. The additional impact of using general anesthesia in people with neurological conditions has not been well studied and adds an unknown risk for people undergoing DBS. Additionally, detection of bleeding in the brain may be difficult during asleep surgery and the overall risk and long-term benefit of asleep DBS surgery is still unknown.

Time in the operating room: Operating room time will depend on the surgical technique and whether the surgery is staged. Your surgeon will inform you and your family of your expected time in the operating room.

Time in the hospital after surgery: You will remain in the hospital for at least one night after the DBS wire is implanted. The length of stay in the hospital depends on your recovery from the surgery. Typical hospital stays of one to three days is common. You may see physical therapy or occupational therapy before you are discharged home. Your hospital stay may be extended if hospital based rehabilitation or if confusion occurs from the surgery, pain medications or general anesthesia.

Neurostimulator (Battery) Insertion: The neurostimulator may be implanted on the day of brain surgery or delayed for a few days or weeks. General anesthesia (asleep) is typical for this procedure. The surgeon will connect your previously implanted DBS wire to an extension wire which then connects to the battery. The battery is generally implanted under the collar bone. You may have one or two DBS batteries depending on your lifestyle, hobbies or personal preferences. All hardware is under the skin.

Practical Tips: The battery placement often causes more soreness with a longer recovery time than the brain surgery. Ice packs can reduce pain and swelling and limit the need for strong pain medicines after the battery insertion. Make sure you keep the area clean and dry per your surgeon's recommendations.

The First Few Days Or Weeks

Stimulation is not typically turned on the first few days or weeks after DBS surgery. Some people experience improvement in their symptoms known as the *honeymoon period* or *micro-lesion effect.* The micro-lesion effect is a temporary improvement in symptoms caused by brain changes associated with the DBS wire placement. The effect is temporary and can last a few days or a few weeks. It is common for people to ask to decrease or discontinue medications during this time. *Reducing medications without medical guidance is very risky and not advised.* The micro-lesion effect typically subsides without warning and symptoms return to your baseline. For your safety, discuss medications with your DBS neurologist after DBS surgery.

Practical Tips: The following is critical to reduce risk of infection:
- ***Do not pull, pick or remove your sutures or scabs.***
- ***Avoid touching the skin where the incisions are located.***
- ***Do not apply any treatment to the incision to include creams, oils or ointments unless directed specifically by your surgeon.***

The First Month

Monitor your skin (look but do not touch) daily for healing and signs of infection. Signs of infection include drainage, redness, swelling, pain or problems with healing. Hardware removal may be required if an infection develops near the DBS hardware. You will have incisions on the scalp, chest and possibly the neck. You will see the surgeon for suture removal within the first two weeks after surgery. Be sure to follow your surgeon's skin care directions during this time to reduce your risk of infection. Avoid harsh soaps or shampoos, creams or ointments as they can impede skin healing. Do not use pre-surgery cleansers on your skin after DBS surgery.

Practical Tips: Ask your surgeon for written skin care recommendations. Call your surgeon if you experience the following: fever, chills, nausea or vomiting, redness, discharge and increase in pain at the incision sites, headache, confusion, sedation, and change in walking, balance, strength or coordination or vision changes.

Incisions typically heal within two to four weeks depending on your skin and general health. People with Parkinson's can have oily skin which may delay healing. *New or worsening redness is an early warning sign for infection.* Check your pillow each morning and report any signs of drainage from the scalp incision to your surgeon. Do not touch incisions or remove your sutures.

POST-SURGERY SAFETY TIPS

This list does not replace your surgeon's recommendations.

- Ask your surgeon for an emergency contact phone number to call in case you have problems.
- Do not change medications without medical advice.
- Call your surgeon and/or neurology team immediately if you experience, signs of infection, new or worsening symptoms after discharge from the hospital such as fever, chills, warmth pain or discharge over incisions, vomiting, headache, excessive sleepiness, confusion, hallucinations, paranoia, mood changes, vision changes, weakness or seizures can indicate life threatening problems.
- Know when you should restart medications you stopped prior to surgery such as blood thinners (i.e. Coumadin, Plavix or aspirin).
- Ask when you can travel, fly, drive, lift heavy objects.
- Follow the written wound care instructions exactly. *DO NOT REMOVE OR PICK AT STERI-STRIPS OR SUTURE TIPS THAT STICK THOUGH THE SKIN.* Call your surgeon if any concerns about your sutures or skin.

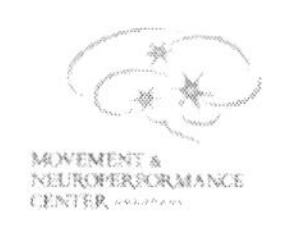

NOTES

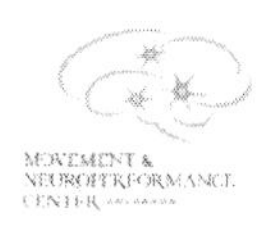

4 STIMULATION ADJUSTMENTS

Your First Programming Appointment

Your first programming session will usually occur two to four weeks after brain surgery to allow the brain time to heal. During this visit, your DBS system will be turned on and stimulation settings will be customized. Be sure to follow instructions provided for this important visit.

There are six main goals in managing your DBS device:

1. Achieve maximal benefit from stimulation.
2. Avoid stimulation induced side effects.
3. Maximize neurostimulator battery life.
4. Monitor hardware integrity and function.
5. Troubleshoot problems.
6. Examine the skin around the device for problems.

Important points related to your first programming appointment are:

- Ask your programmer if you should change your medication for the first adjustment appointment. You should not change your medications without consulting with your medical provider.
- Bring your patient programmer.
- Bring someone with you for support and to take notes.
- Bring medications, cane, walker or wheelchair for balance.
- Reserve up to 2-4 hours for your first programming session.
- Comfort suggestions: wear comfortable clothing that allows for easy examination of the neck and chest incision site; bring a warm jacket, snack, water, book, magazine, and/or family or friend to share in the experience.
- Mention if you noticed drainage or redness around the incision.
- Report changes in thinking, walking, swallowing or mood.

Deep brain stimulation is an adjustable therapy and there are a variety of techniques used to reach the above goals. During the first appointment, your medical provider will activate your device and test several settings to find the best therapeutic effect.

A structured approach during the first stimulation appointment provides a valuable framework to guide future stimulation adjustments. This approach reduces side effects and the time required to adjust the neurostimulator at subsequent programming visits.

The first programming session is typically scheduled two to four weeks after electrode implantation to allow time for the *microlesion effect* to subside and may also occur off medication. This strategy helps ensure your symptoms are present and can be measured while the stimulation is adjusted so your programmer can discover optimal stimulation settings.

Customizing Stimulation

Each brain target has predictable stimulation settings if the lead wire is well placed in the target. The location of the electrodes determine the maximal intensity of stimulation that is possible. Spreading stimulation beyond the brain target will result in side effects unless the intensity is reduced. Just a quick glance at the relative size of each brain target conforms with the typical stimulation settings customarily applied to each target.

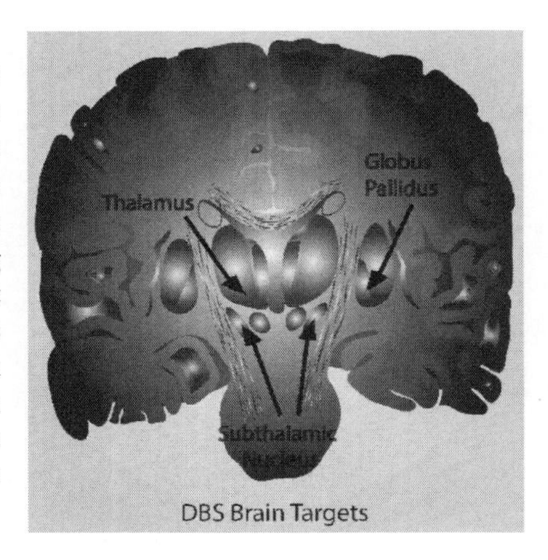

DBS Brain Targets

Your hardware system is checked first before beginning each programming session to check your neurostimulator battery status and to confirm wires are not damaged and electrical pulses are reaching the brain.

The primary goal of the first programming is to activate (turn on) the best electrode that will provide you with the most benefit. **Stimulation should work as expected if the following conditions are met:**

- patient has the right diagnosis
- DBS is done at the right time
- Lead wire is implanted in the right location
- stimulation is adjusted properly
- hardware is intact.

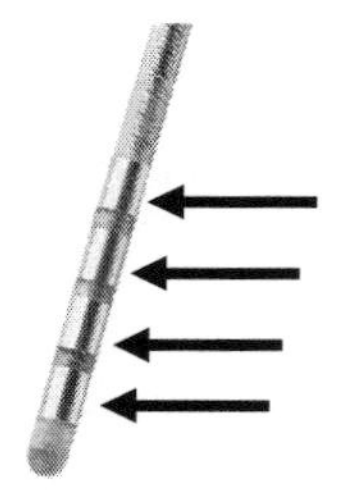
4 Electrode Bands are available to activate as negative or positive

The wire has four electrodes stacked together at the tip. Stimulation can be focused around each electrode independently, allowing the programmer to customize where the stimulation is focused within the target. Ideally, each electrode is tested using increasing voltages until maximal benefit is noted and stimulation side effects are recorded. Benefit and side effects depend on the exact location of your electrodes. This collective procedure is called *electrode mapping.* Common and expected stimulation side effects include tingling, lightheadedness, muscle twitching or contraction and speech changes. All stimulation side effects are reversible. Clarifying which settings cause stimulation side effects is a very important step to fully understand the limits of your DBS and prevent stimulation related problems. When stimulation intensity is reduced, the side effect will subside. **Optimal and effective stimulation settings do not cause stimulation side effects or pain as long as the electrode is well positioned in the desired brain target and stimulation is set appropriately.** (See chapter 5.)

Once your electrodes are mapped (detection of benefit and side effects), your medical provider will select the best settings for your symptoms. Typically, one or sometimes two of the four electrodes are perfectly located in the brain target. Settings are chosen to focus stimulation around these electrodes that provide the best response. Activating an *ineffective* electrode will limit benefit, can result in quick loss of benefit after the adjustment or cause bothersome stimulation side effects.

You will see or feel symptoms improve within seconds to minutes after turning on the stimulation. Muscle stiffness and tremor improve quickly and are useful measures of whether stimulation is helping. Dyskinesia, slowness, shuffling and dystonia improve more slowly with stimulation and may take many weeks or months for optimal results. The first programming session is usually time intensive. Plan for up to three hours; however the time may vary depending on the preferences of your medical provider.

Stimulation Parameters Can Be Adjusted

The following stimulation parameters are adjusted to maximize benefit:

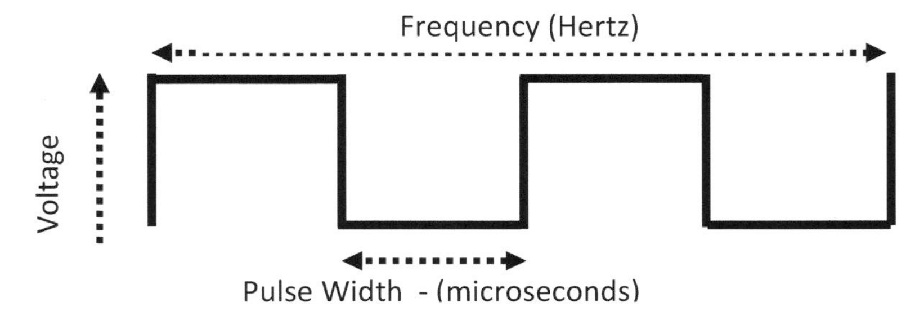

- **Electrode Activation**: The electrode that provides the most benefit is set as the negative (cathode). The negative electrode produces the greatest impact for improving symptoms but if selected poorly, can result in inducing stimulation side effects or no effect. Activating a positive (anode) electrode condenses the spread of electric current and is a strategy used to avoid side effects.

- **Voltage (volts):** an increase in voltage increases the intensity (amount of tissue stimulated) adjacent to the negative electrode. Constant current is not discussed but is an option to use to adjust intensity. The principles are the same whether using volts or amps.

- **Pulse Width (microseconds):** the time the pulse lingers in the tissue.

- **Frequency (hertz):** (pulses per second) the effective frequencies typically range from 130 to 185 hertz.

- **Polarity (monopolar or bipolar):** describes electrode configuration such as whether electrodes are activated as negative or positive. Polarity further shapes (customizes) the area of stimulation. The polarity illustration shows the difference in monopolar and bipolar.

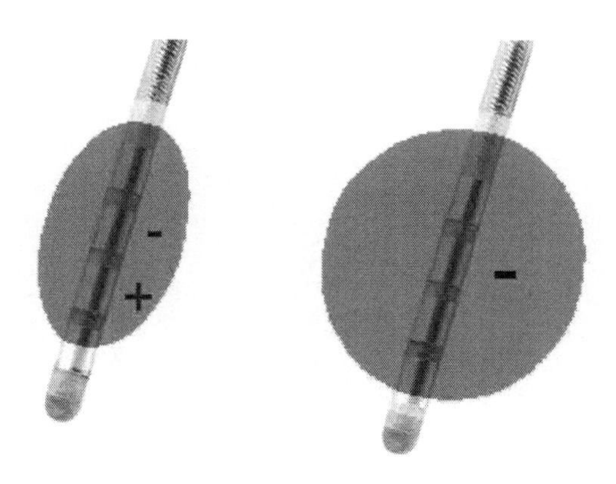

Bipolar vs Monopolar

Stimulation parameters are adjusted to maximize benefit and battery longevity while avoiding side effects. Your neurostimulator can be programmed so you can change stimulation at home using settings determined while in the clinic and deemed safe for you when not under medical supervision.

Timeline for Improvement

The time-line is a generalization and depends on your diagnosis, symptoms, medications and preferences of the medical clinician.

Deep brain stimulation is known to improve movement symptoms and may result in less reliance on medication. Research data shows that DBS benefits can last up to 10 years. Our clinical experience suggests that DBS continues to work well beyond 10 years and is superior to medication alone. Knowing what to expect each month after DBS can alleviate worries and fears that the DBS may or may not be working. The timeline below is a general description of what to expect (although this can vary) after stimulation is turned on.

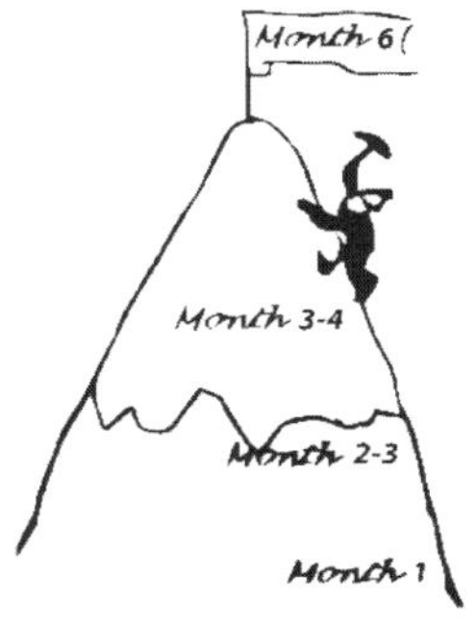

Month 1: This is your brain's introduction to stimulation. During month one, stimulation intensity may be low and medication reduction can be limited depending on the severity of your symptoms. Dyskinesia can result from stimulation and unlike medicine induced dyskinesia, stimulation induced dyskinesia is considered a positive predictor for good results. Dyskinesia typically subsides within days to weeks or can be managed with slower voltage increases and medication reduction.

Month 2 to 3: You are starting to feel better with less need for medication, less dyskinesia, less dystonia, less tremor and overall more *on time*. Until final stimulation intensity is reached, your benefit can still diminish between appointments and this is a common time-frame to feel frustrated if improvement is less than you expected. Patience is important as the brain needs time to accommodate stimulation and build the foundation for sustained improvement in symptoms. Individuals with tremor may have obtained optimal improvement by the third month.

> What activities can improve after DBS? Dexterity, eating, drinking, rolling over in bed, standing up, getting in and out of a car, getting dressed, walking longer distances, exercise, length and quality of sleep, pain, outlook, going out socially, shopping and quality of living. Recent reports indicate DBS may extend life in people with PD.

Month 4 to 5: Stimulation settings are now close to being optimized, medication dosages are being reduced. You are feeling like DBS was a good decision and the beneficial effects last longer between appointments. Individuals with dystonia should be noticing some benefit in pain, abnormal posturing, and tremor.

Month 6: By month six, *on time*, tremor or dystonia is significantly improved and the beneficial effects noted in clinic do not wear off between visits. Little change is required over the next 6 months. After six to twelve months, you may require little to no change in your stimulation settings until you need your DBS battery replaced.

Stimulation and Medication

If you have Parkinson's disease, your first programming is typically performed off medication when symptoms are obvious. Since medication and stimulation interact, you will likely be asked to take your medication after stimulation is adjusted to observe the combined effect. The additive effects can result in too much movement (dyskinesia) or feeling of overstimulation. When medications start to take effect, the stimulation intensity can easily be reduced before you leave the clinic if you feel overstimulated or develop bothersome dyskinesia.

Your response to stimulation with medication will be a factor in the selection of your stimulation settings. Although medications can be reduced to counteract overstimulation or dyskinesia, safety is top priority. If significant dyskinesia, motor fluctuations, balance, falling or walking is a concern, stimulation intensity may be increased slowly to allow the brain time to accommodate. Medications can then be reduced once there is a solid foundation of stimulation to buffer the effects of less medication.

Unlike *medication* induced dyskinesia, *stimulation* induced dyskinesia will typically fade over time. If dyskinesia is a significant problem, stimulation adjustments may take a little longer to avoid injury from severe or ballistic movements. Medication reduction may be an earlier priority in the process if dyskinesia is bothersome after stimulation is activated.

Adjusting stimulation to reach the final setting is like a marathon, steady and deliberate progress will get you to the finish line. Adjusting stimulation and medications is based on the experience and preferences of your neurologist and tailored to the individual. In the next section we review some specific differences for each diagnosis approved for DBS.

Parkinson's disease. The majority of people with PD continue to require medication after DBS. Medication reduction, however, is common and may depend on the brain target and the specific symptoms you are experiencing. As stimulation improves *on* time, less medication is needed throughout the day and night. Stimulation effects are typically optimized the first four to six months after surgery. Medication reduction is in part based on whether you are experiencing dyskinesia, off periods, mobility problems, non-motor symptoms such as depression or medication side effects such as sedation or thinking difficulties.

Tremor. Tremor responds quickly to stimulation within minutes but may take a few months to see the full effect. The figure on the right illustrates an initial stimulation adjustment and the noted improvement in spiral drawing as the voltage is increased. Medications can be reduced and sometimes stopped if tremor is the predominant problem. This must be done slowly even if your tremor improves dramatically. Reducing medicine too quickly can cause withdrawal symptoms. Some tremor medications are also used to treat blood pressure, pain, mood or seizures. Discuss any change in medication with your prescribing physician.

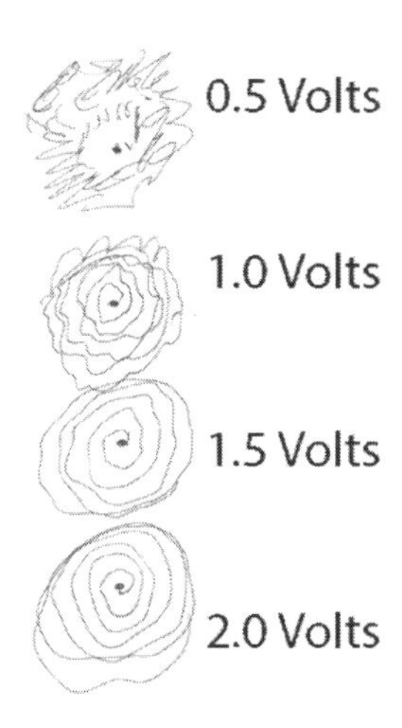

Dystonia. Dystonic symptoms can take longer to respond to stimulation, sometimes up to a year before symptoms are greatly improved. Your response to stimulation will guide medication decisions. Medication reduction is possible as dystonic contractions and pain improves with stimulation but changes made too rapidly can result in a dystonic crisis, insomnia, muscle pain, discomfort, confusion and anxiety.

Subsequent Programming Visits and Long Term Care

Initial changes in stimulation settings typically occur every two to four weeks for PD and tremor and less often for dystonia. Ask your medical provider about *how many visits* to expect the first year. *Be patient.* You may need three to six months to optimize your deep brain stimulation treatment. Do not expect your symptoms to improve immediately. Improvement takes time and cannot be rushed. Too much and too rapid an increase in stimulation can cause stimulation side effects. Knowing that progress takes time will reduce un-necessary worry.

Your DBS system can be turned on and off. For best response, keep DBS on at all times if you have Parkinson's or dystonia. You can turn DBS off at night if you have tremor but DBS can be left on if tremor is bothersome while you are trying to sleep. Learn how to use your *patient programmer* in case you need to adjust or turn off your stimulation.

Weight gain is possible following STN DBS surgery. Exercise should become part of your routine after surgery. More information on exercise and nutrition is available in chapter 7. Physical therapy, occupational therapy and speech therapy may be part of your post-operative care to optimize your functional outcome of surgery.

Practical Tips: Wear a helmet during any risky activities and report any head trauma to your neurologist since this may damage DBS wires. ID Cards are issued by the device company. Keep your contact information up to date with the device company.

As a patient, you may be asking your neurologist or programmer over the months and years to increase stimulation to improve symptoms. An experienced programmer will help you understand when it is appropriate to change stimulation settings. One way to avoid overstimulation side effects is to remember what DBS can and cannot do (read the first two chapters of this book as a refresher). The following tips help avoid overstimulation:

- DBS is not a cure. Symptoms that do not respond to stimulation may require medication or rehabilitation.
- Stimulation side effects will occur if stimulation exceeds the boundaries of the intended brain target. There is a maximum limit of stimulation that will be tolerated. Since the brain region stimulated does not grow larger in size over time, maximum limits in stimulation do not increase over time.
  - Disease progression is a factor that may prompt you to request a change in settings. This is especially true for Parkinson's disease. Balance, freezing of gait, speech, and swallowing problems are examples of symptoms that worsen and do not usually improve with stimulation. Increasing stimulation for disease progression is a common cause of overstimulation induced side effects.
- If you have not experienced the expected benefit over the first six to twelve months, you may require additional appointments to troubleshoot why DBS is not working as expected.

Practical Tips: Stimulation side effects can cause worsening of symptoms such as walking, balance, swallowing and speech. Inform your neurologist about any abrupt change in these symptoms.

LONG-TERM CARE PHASE

Long-term follow-up visits include a careful examination of your skin around the battery and scalp. The skin that is directly over the hardware can become thin. This may require surgery so that the battery or wires do not erode through the skin. This is not common but can occur in older, thin or malnourished individuals. Your hardware system is also checked for problems and battery life is noted at each visit. Call your neurologist immediately if you notice redness or skin irritation around the DBS battery or wires, experience tingling, heat sensation, shocks or pain around the neurostimulator or wires or a change in mood.

DBS and Non-Motor Symptoms in Parkinson's

Rapid medicine reduction may cause or worsen depression, anxiety and apathy. It is not clear if depression is best treated with standard medications such as antidepressants or an increase in PD medications. Increasing PD medications may be necessary, in the short-term to treat any emergence of anxiety or depression after DBS. Suicide has been reported to occur after DBS and, in most cases, was unexpected occurring without pre-existing depression. Reporting fluctuations in mood to your doctor, especially after a stimulation or medication adjustment is important for your safety.

AVOIDING SIDE EFFECTS

Excessive or inappropriate stimulation can cause side effects just like excessive or inappropriate use of medication can cause side effects. Stimulation induced side effects are **reversible** and can include *muscle contraction or twitching, eye closure, muscle tightness, slowness, change in coordination, speech changes, sense of muscle heaviness, staggering, balance changes, walking changes* (leg dragging, stumbling, freezing) tingling, numbness, dizziness, pulsations, surges, wave sensations, vision changes, mood changes or cognitive changes (mental fog). Side effects occur when stimulation spreads beyond the intended brain target. Reducing stimulation intensity can alleviate side effects. Stimulation intensity is controlled by polarity, voltage and pulse width. The drawing (page 62) shows the difference in stimulation intensity when using monopolar versus bipolar polarity. The gray oval represents a typical area (spread) of stimulation in the brain tissue when using either bipolar or monopolar. Monopolar (negative electrode only) induces a large area of stimulation around the electrode. If used properly, symptoms respond well without side effects. However, if side effects are limiting benefit, bipolar polarity and minimal pulse width is commonly used to reduce the spread of stimulation. Final stimulation settings ultimately depend on the location of the electrodes in the brain target.

Troubleshooting Less Than Expected Results

Troubleshooting may be required if symptoms have not improved as expected or if there is an abrupt loss of benefit. Sometimes there are clues why DBS is not working but often a more extensive evaluation must be done. Few centers have DBS troubleshooting clinics to determine the cause of loss of therapy or poor outcome. Troubleshooting clinics often require several visits to investigate problems. Sometimes, more than one issue (listed below) can impact outcomes.

Misplaced electrodes	Hardware damage	Medicine dose too low
Inappropriate stimulation settings	Incorrect diagnosis	Unrealistic expectations

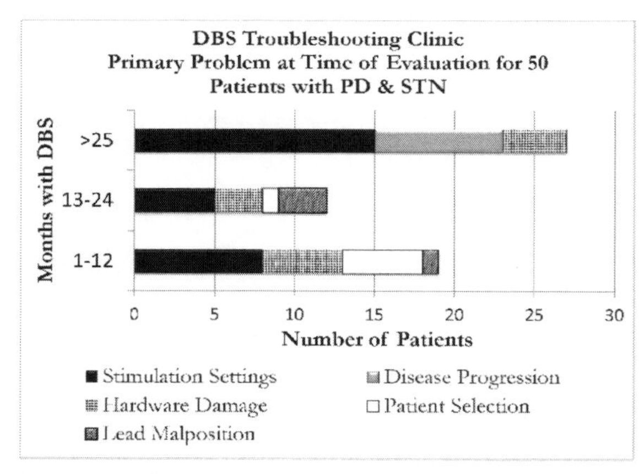

The graph illustrates reasons for poor outcome as analyzed in the author's troubleshooting clinic. Whether immediately after surgery or many years thereafter, the predominant problem was inadequate or inappropriate stimulation settings reinforcing the need for a skilled team. Source: *Retrospective Review of Factors Leading to Dissatisfaction with STN DBS during Long-term Management.* Published in Surgical Neurology International by Farris S, Giroux ML. June 2013, 4-69.
(Graph modified for this publication, article available DBSGuide.com.)

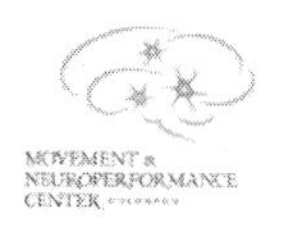

NOTES

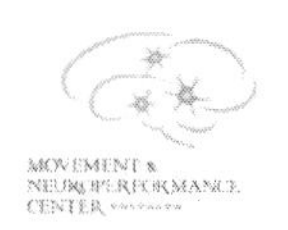

5 TROUBLESHOOTING

"I wouldn't call what I do a job – it's more of a passion. For years I have had the privilege to witness the power and joy of DBS as time seems to go in reverse and symptoms melt away. When DBS doesn't work or causes problems, I can feel the distress and hopelessness of my patients. I am truly driven to investigate and solve problems when DBS fails. Most often, problems or failed benefit can be better understood and turned around with a methodical analysis. We owe our patients a second or third look when such a powerful therapy fails to deliver."

-Sierra Farris PA-C

When Results are Less Than Expected

There are situations in which the outcome is less than desired and DBS troubleshooting may be necessary. Troubleshooting requires a structured evaluation designed to identify the cause or factor(s) that contribute to patient dissatisfaction or poor results. The most common cause(s) for poor results or dissatisfaction include:

1. *Diagnosis.* Parkinson's disease, essential tremor and primary dystonia respond best to DBS and reported benefits are based on these neurologic conditions. Other conditions that mimic PD, tremor or dystonia are not likely to respond to DBS and may worsen after DBS surgery. Avoid poor results by confirming your diagnosis. On-off medicine testing for Parkinson's and a careful neurologic assessment of tremor and dystonia can help confirm your diagnosis and discuss the expected results from surgery.

2. *Electrode placement.* DBS electrodes must be implanted with millimeter precision for best results. Brain imaging and electrode mapping in the clinic can help determine if lead wires were accurately placed during surgery.

3. *Stimulation Settings.* Stimulation should be confined to the area that provides benefit and avoids side effects. If stimulation intensity is too high, stimulation can spread beyond the brain target and cause serious side effects. This is the most common source of poor outcomes.

4. *DBS system damage.* Hardware can break and the wire insulation can become damaged. Your medical provider can check your wires and battery at each visit to insure your system is intact.

5. *Disease Progression.* As disease progresses, troublesome symptoms can emerge that will not respond to stimulation. This is especially true for Parkinson's disease. A review of your specific problems and *on-off* medicine testing can help determine symptoms that should respond to stimulation. This is a common cause for dissatisfaction with DBS over time.

6. *Medication and other non-DBS therapy.* You may still need medication and other therapies such as rehabilitation. Reducing medication too much or failing to change medicine with stimulation can result in additional problems of over or under dosing.

7. *Patient and family expectations.* Patients and their families may expect DBS to improve symptoms that are not responsive to DBS. Examples include balance, freezing of gait, speech and swallowing problems. The more a symptom affects your life, the more you may pursue stimulation adjustments to improve these symptoms. Be sure to review the *Expectation & Symptom Worksheet* in chapter 1 to be sure your expectations are aligned with what DBS can improve. (Note: As you will learn below, overstimulation can also cause these problems and this must be differentiated from disease progression.)

The following story was written by a patient that underwent DBS troubleshooting after experiencing poor results from DBS. He knew his situation was atypical however he encountered difficulty finding solutions. His story reveals the importance of finding a team that *listens* and the critical need for patients to become highly knowledgeable about DBS and advocate for the best possible care.

Dean's Journey

In every life there comes a defining moment. One that alters the landscape in a permanent way. Mine came 17 years ago-at age 40-while I was sitting in a chair quietly reading. My little finger began to dance as if it were hearing its own music. I had no idea my mind was beginning to compose a personal musical score. My body became the blank pages with the notes, tempo, and rhythm inked in by my brain. I was simply a conduit for this process, never asked for my input as the composition choreographed my body's movements. It took four years for the score to reveal its title: Parkinson's disease. From a musical perspective, Parkinson's comes in variations, with unique styles and tempos, and a melody that differs from person to person. Our bodies move to their own changing rhythms that we must adapt to.

Facing the music. *For years my symptoms have been managed with the traditional Parkinson's drugs. Because the disease's symptoms are progressive and ever-changing, the drug treatment is often a lot of trial and error. I have been under-medicated. I've also been overmedicated. Like a silent thief, Parkinson's has stolen from me over the years. I had built a home, supporting myself as an artist and blacksmith. Baking pies and breads to sell at the local farmers market was also a means of support. Playing banjo, piano, and other instruments, as well as restoring vintage cars occupied any spare moments.*

'A new lease on life.' *Over time, my unpredictable, but increasingly frequent, off periods incapacitated and exhausted me. My social interactions and ability to venture out into the world began to shrink as my time was spent anticipating and managing symptoms. A true miracle occurred during these dark days. I fell in love with Jennifer, a lovely and truly amazing woman. Jennifer's caring embodies unconditional love, and our life together is filled with laughter and joy despite Parkinson's and everything in its wake. Jennifer supported my decision to undergo deep brain stimulation (DBS) surgery. My doctors had suggested I was a good candidate for the procedure, and it seemed the logical—if not the only—option left to improve my quality of life. My frustrations with the disease had become greater than my reluctance to undergo my third open-head procedure, and I scheduled surgery.*

A disappointing reality. *From all reports my surgery went perfectly, and I went home with high expectations. An appointment was scheduled with my neurologist, who would determine which settings would give me the greatest relief with the fewest side effects. I was flirting with disappointment when I left this first session with my voice weakened and swallowing felt strange. But I kept the faith my body would adjust.*

But the outcome of each monthly session seemed to follow a pattern. Benefits achieved with a new setting disappeared within days. When I expressed concern about my nearly inaudible voice and difficulty swallowing, I was referred to speech therapy. At the same time my left side was becoming weaker and dexterity was disappearing in my left hand and arm, rendering it mostly useless. My Parkinson's symptoms seemed to be accelerating at a very rapid pace. Because my tremors would increase when the DBS device was turned off, there was continual reassurance that the procedure was working, and I continued to hold to the hope that the right adjustment would be made. Eventually I was told the programmer had found the optimum settings for me.

By this point, carrying on conversations was all but futile since my voice was so soft that nobody could hear me. Eating and drinking were becoming more and more uncomfortable and dangerous as my swallowing reflex was weak and unreliable. I could barely use my left hand or arm, so operating a computer was extremely difficult. I used a wheelchair to get around but needed to be pushed since my left side was so weak. I was mentally and physically exhausted each moment of every day. I questioned the doctors about what else might be done for me. Eventually, my doctor looked me in the eye and told me I needed to face the fact that I had advanced Parkinson's and learn to live with it. Everything changed for me that afternoon. The lights went off and the darkness covered me with a cloak of blackness so thick and deep I could not see. The one thing that had kept me going—hope—had been taken away.

Getting it back. Running in the background here is another story. My sister, a big believer in options, had discovered a DBS program specialized in troubleshooting disappointing outcomes such as mine. This team listened to my story, evaluated my programming, checking each electrode systematically for benefits and side effects and performed brain imaging. The results were clear. My speech, swallowing and walking problems were not disease progression. I was experiencing side effects because the leads were not in the right place and stimulation outside of the intended STN target was causing these problems.

A new dance. Several weeks later we sat in the neurosurgeon's office discussing another surgery to remove and reposition the electrode on the right side of my brain, which controlled the left side of my body. And though I was agreeing to open-head surgery number four, I had absolutely no second thoughts. Jennifer and I couldn't stop smiling as we drove home filled with hope.

It was a new experience for me to be greeted with excitement at a medical appointment, but a month later it was palpable as I sat with my programmer for my programming visit. Today, seven months later, I have no apparent tremor and my body is quiet. I can walk, talk, drive a car, and undertake many of the projects I never thought I'd be able to do again. Each morning as I stroll through the woods near our home, resting on the walking stick I recently carved from a fallen branch, I reflect on my journey.

My medical team gave me back my life. I leave each visit with better understanding and a greater feeling of control. Perhaps best of all was the realization that someone in the medical community saw me as a human being. I hadn't been listened to in such a long time that I'd forgotten what it was like to be heard.

The musical score that my body continues to compose will always be called Parkinson's disease—but these days I often enjoy the music. Today it may be a waltz, tomorrow a two-step. But whatever the dance, I do it with joy.
-Dean Crumpacker

Troubleshooting Analysis of Dean's DBS Outcome[1]

Dean's story illustrates the many factors that ultimately affect outcomes. Dean had DBS at the right time; not too early and not too late. His diagnosis, symptoms and reason for pursuing surgery were ideal as was his expectation and goal to reduce off time, decrease medication and improve tremor, slowness, stiffness and shuffling. Yet, Dean had experienced great declines in his mobility, speech and swallowing. He was using a wheelchair, considering a feeding tube and feared he was facing a nursing home.

We reviewed his medical history. There were no red flags for Dean to undergo DBS surgery. He was young, had PD for 11 years and his expectation that tremor and on-time would improve was appropriate. His surgery went well without complications and the recovery from DBS was uneventful.

Once stimulation was initiated, new symptoms appeared and old symptoms were getting worse. Most importantly, Dean was not getting better. Improvement is seen within the first year of surgery yet Dean was worse not better. Additional tests were performed in effort to diagnose the cause of the new problems. His new diagnosis-disease progression.

When he contacted us for a second opinion, he had DBS for 19 months. We reviewed Dean's brain scans, and noticed a possible problem with his right DBS lead that appeared to be outside the typical area of the STN. This was confirmed during his programming evaluation.

---

[1] Dean Crumpacker provided permission to include the details of his troubleshooting evaluation.

On Dean's first day of troubleshooting, we examined him before making any changes to his stimulation and once again after turning stimulation off. Off stimulation, Dean's tremor worsened but speech, motivation, facial expression, balance, slowness, walking, and hand movements improved. Our suspicion was confirmed; Dean suffered from stimulation side effects that mimicked disease progression.

The next step was a two hour process that included a detailed analysis of benefit and side effects for each electrode to analyze which settings were causing problems and whether stimulation settings could be changed to improve benefit.

The left DBS lead was working well but the right DBS lead was not accurately placed and causing stimulation side effects. Dean required another surgery to remove and replace the right lead. With the new right lead in the correct location, stimulation gave Dean the results he expected. Dean now lives with the benefit he expected and is not deteriorating from stimulation side effects. The following section further reviews these and other common problems or difficulties that can occur at different time points after surgery.

First Few Weeks After Surgery

Complications can be seen immediately after DBS surgery and are thought to be due to brain changes associated with the surgery, the stress of surgery and/or general anesthesia. The following symptoms and problems can emerge within the first few hours, days, weeks or months after surgery.

A decline in verbal fluency or change in language skills can be observed. This is described as a difficulty finding the correct words during conversation or problems making a complete sentence. Verbal fluency is just one aspect of cognition but an important component that is at risk of declining due to the surgical procedure. Verbal fluency is measured during the pre-surgical neuropsychological evaluation and these results are a very important part of the pre-surgery evaluation. If verbal fluency is poor before surgery there is greater risk of problems after DBS.

Confusion, psychosis, personality change, extreme fatigue or sleepiness are other potential cognitive complications caused by the surgical procedure, bleeding in the brain, general anesthesia or pain medications prescribed after surgery. Cognitive changes are usually temporary and resolve as the brain heals over the first few months. Permanent and troublesome cognitive changes after surgery are uncommon if cognitive abilities were strong prior to surgery.

Walking and balance problems can occur, albeit uncommon, as a result of *surgery*. Bleeding in the brain is a known risk during surgery and can cause stroke symptoms that include walking or balance changes. Lastly, there is a rare chance of permanent walking problems after DBS surgery even before stimulation is turned on. This is uncommon, not understood and unpredictable at this time.

Potential Complications – First Six to Twelve Months

Stimulation settings are customized during the *optimization phase*. Typically symptoms will improve as stimulation is optimized and then plateau over a period of twelve months. When settings are optimal, little change will be required over the subsequent years. Improvement should be noted along with medicine reduction. Inadequate stimulation settings, misplaced electrodes or wire damage and incorrect diagnosis are common reasons why DBS goals are not met during the first year.

Practical Tips: Stimulation is optimized the first 12 months after surgery. If symptoms do not improve during the first 6 to 12 months, further exploration may be needed to identify the reason(s) why.

Potential Complications – Long-term DBS Therapy

Once optimization is complete, the next phase in DBS care is the *maintenance phase*. During this time, medication doses continue to be streamlined, your neurostimulator battery is monitored and hardware system is checked to make sure everything remains intact and functioning. During the maintenance phase, any sudden loss of therapy can be caused by a low or depleted neurostimulator battery, wire damage, inappropriate change in stimulation settings, and significant change in medicines or turning off the neurostimulator. A gradual decline in symptoms in the absence of stimulation change often suggests disease progression, an undetected wire problem or depleting battery.

Disease Progression

Disease progression in PD is associated with a gradual decline in speech, swallowing, balance or walking problems. As you have learned, inappropriate stimulation settings, inadequate positioning of the electrodes or drastic medication reduction can also be the cause. Worsening mobility should prompt a thorough investigation into stimulation settings, medication dosing, electrode location and disease progression since declines in mobility jeopardize independence and can lead to injury from falls.

Answer the questions below to help you and your team determine if any of the scenarios outlined below are a cause of your problem.

When did speech, walking or balance problems begin?

1. before DBS or within the first year after DBS?
2. after a change in stimulation settings and/or a change in medications?
3. after a new medical problem that could explain the walking and/or balance symptoms?
4. after a new medication was added to your regimen?
5. many years after DBS?

Problems Old and New

A Sudden & New Problem: If walking or balance problems are new after DBS surgery, it is important to be sure your *medication dose* is adequate. Medication reduction after DBS is expected but the speed of reduction will vary. Safe medication reduction depends on your sense of stability, baseline balance, physical health and fitness. Another cause of new onset mobility problems is inappropriate *stimulation.* Stimulation induced side effects of leg dragging, gait freezing, gait slowness, staggering, spontaneous falling, foot drop, toe dragging or loss of postural control can occur from over-stimulation, inadequate stimulation settings or poor electrode position within the brain. These scenarios are illustrated in the following pages and are reversible causes of mobility problems.

An Old Problem that is Rapidly Getting Worse: Sudden changes in mobility are typically tracked back to an event, such as an illness, fall, medication or stimulation change. A *fall* or accident can result in *damage* to the DBS hardware system and this can cause a sudden worsening of mobility. A check to insure the system is working is important in the setting of an acute loss of therapy or worsening symptoms, especially after a fall.

Stimulation side effects should be investigated if walking and/or balance problems suddenly become worse. Stimulation induced mobility side effects may be accompanied by other stimulation side effects that include speech slurring or volume loss, facial spasm, swallowing problems, dizziness, blurred or double vision, visual wave phenomenon, tingling, numbness, surge sensation, slowness of movement, mood change or mental fog, muscle tightness or a new tremor.

An Old Problem that is Slowly Getting Worse: Walking and balance requires complex control that involves multiple intact neurological and orthopedic systems. Changes in walking and balance are expected with Parkinson's and may be present in people with tremor, dystonia or with aging. Gradual change in mobility is seen with disease progression. Other problems common with aging can also contribute including peripheral neuropathy, diabetes, vision loss, vitamin B12 deficiency, hypothyroidism, joint pain, stroke, spine problems and cognitive declines are common causes for walking and/or balance changes as we age. These problems when coupled with the Parkinson's, tremor or dystonia, can cause additional balance problems or mobility difficulties.

A Holistic Treatment Approach

A comprehensive care approach will enhance your life quality after DBS. As we have discussed throughout this book, doing your best also requires a balance of medical, rehabilitative, emotional and lifestyle changes. There is a tendency to look to DBS to improve all problems and forget about the many other factors and treatments important for your wellbeing. Remember DBS is only one aspect of your therapy. As Parkinson's, tremor or dystonia progresses, it is important to resist the urge to increase stimulation intensity beyond the threshold for benefit to avoid over-stimulation side effects that can directly worsen walking, balance and speech. Living with stimulation side effects can directly impact your wellbeing after DBS. The following examples review the anatomy and most common side effects associated with overstimulation of the STN.

Stimulation Side Effects – The STN Example

The STN is nestled in the brain between sensation nerve tracts and motor control nerve tracts (see figure below for STN size and location compared to other DBS brain targets). When stimulation spreads into adjacent nerve tracts, side effects will occur. When sensation nerve tracts are stimulated, the person will feel tingling, numbness, surges and sometimes pain. When the motor control nerves are stimulated, normal movement is inhibited causing slurred speech, facial twitching or muscle tightness, contraction, swallowing problems, leg dragging, slow movement, dizziness, wave sensation, vision changes and potentially pain. Below the STN is the substantia nigra and structures that control eye movements. Stimulating below the STN can cause double vision, staggering, falls, sweating, slowness, warm sensations, and Parkinson's medications may work less effectively.

The following scenarios illustrate the relationship between stimulation settings and side effects. Only the STN is reviewed, however the GPi and VIM can be associated with similar side effects. The illustrations are presented in one dimensional format for ease of understanding the neuroanatomy. The top figure (STN close-up) illustrates the relationship between electrode location, stimulation intensity and adjacent structures next to the STN. Electrode placement varies and is customized during surgery. Note that the dark area (sphere) around the active electrode shows the magnitude or region of stimulation around the negative (darkest) electrode. When applying the proper intensity (voltage, pulse width), stimulation is limited to the target and does not over-flow into adjacent areas. Confining the spread of stimulation offers therapeutic benefit without side effects. The second figure illustrates what occurs when an incorrect electrode is activated. In this scenario, there are three electrodes inside the STN yet an electrode outside the STN (darkest) is activated creating an area of stimulation outside the STN. This could result in little to no benefit and/or cause side effects. The goal is to increase stimulation to maximal benefit while avoiding side effects. The bottom figure shows intense stimulation caused by setting the voltage too high (overstimulation). Stimulation spreads into adjacent regions to cause stimulation side effects such as slurred speech, leg

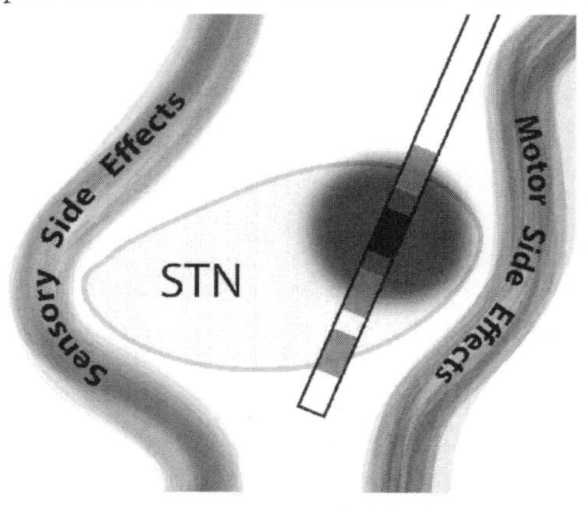

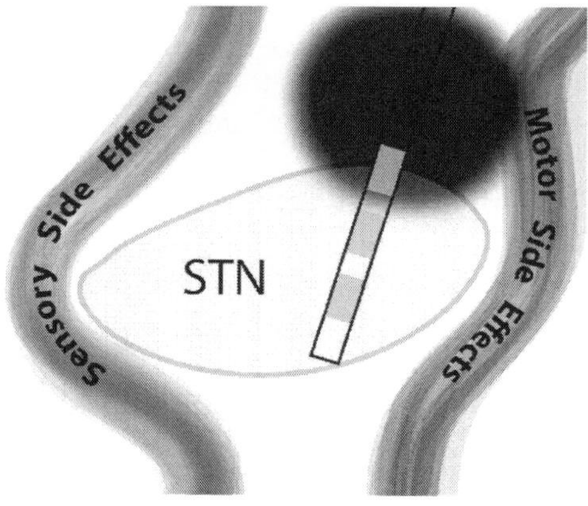

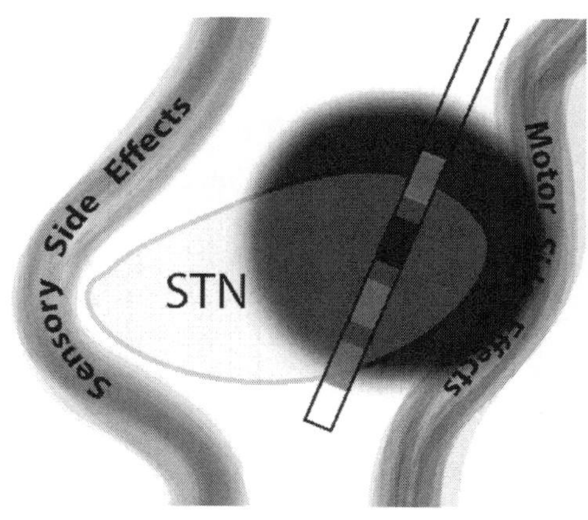

dragging or muscle tightness. Reducing stimulation intensity can eliminate side effects in this example.

The top figure illustrates electrodes that are too close to the sensation nerve tract. When stimulation spreads into this area, side effects can include tingling, numbness, surges as well as imbalance, vision changes and sensation of warmth. If stimulation intensity is limited due to electrode placement or by side effects, a brain scan (MRI or CT scan) can be helpful in determining the location of the electrodes and whether surgery is required to reposition the lead. The final figure on the right illustrates electrodes that are placed too close to the motor control tract. When stimulation spreads into the motor control fibers, side effects of slurred speech, muscle twitching, muscle contraction, pain, dizziness, leg dragging, vision changes, swallowing problems, slow movement, gait freezing or imbalance can occur. In this example, beneficial stimulation cannot be achieved due to poor position of the electrodes and side effects. Repositioning of the wire is needed to achieve beneficial stimulation without side effects.

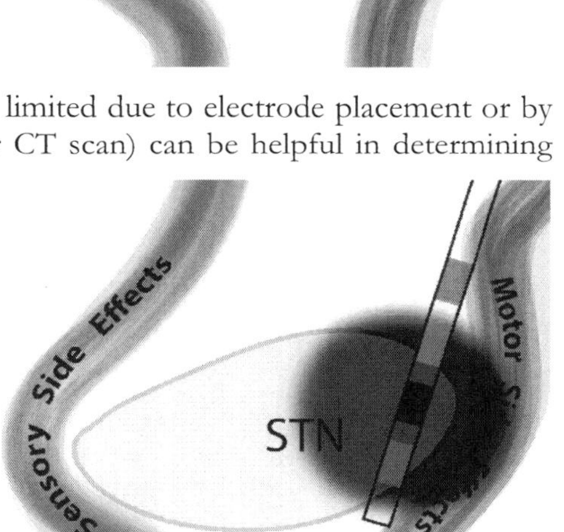

HARDWARE COMPLICATIONS

Hardware problems can occur with any implanted system. The rate of hardware complications vary across centers and are difficult if not impossible to anticipate. The following list includes the most common hardware complications:

1. Sudden loss of power from a depleted battery
2. Wire migration
3. Fluid leakage

4. Skin erosion around hardware
5. Wire kinking, breakage or fraying

Depleted neurostimulator. Your neurostimulator can be checked at each appointment to minimize risk of a sudden loss of power. Your patient programmer also allows you to monitor battery status. Battery life varies and ranges on average from 3 to 4 years. High stimulation intensity or a stimulation technique called *interleaving* will deplete your neurostimulator battery quicker. A short circuit can also deplete your neurostimulator battery at a rapid rate. Routine hardware check-ups help avoid unexpected battery depletion and informs the medical provider of any wire problems.

Wire migration. Wire migration is not common and is diagnosed when the wire moves from the intended location and can typically be seen on a plain skull x-ray. Migration can occur during surgery or as a consequence of

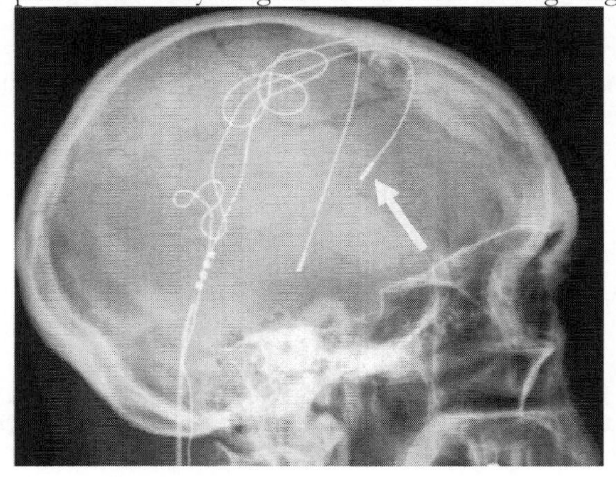

cap malfunctions or if the cap is not closed adequately (the cap covers the small hole in the scalp and secures the wire). Migration can also occur when significant tension pulls on the wire such as after traumatic falls. Wire migration requires additional brain surgery to correct if the electrodes are too far from the target and stimulation is not effective. The x-ray shows migration where the wire moved well above the intended brain target (noted by the arrow).

Fluid leakage. Fluid leakage into hardware connections is uncommon. If fluid leaks into the hardware connections, therapy may not be as effective or a short circuit may be noted during hardware check-ups. This is most common immediately after surgery and often resolves with time. The need for surgical intervention is uncommon.

Skin erosion. Skin erosion is a long-term complication that can lead to infection if not noticed and corrected. Older, thin or malnourished individuals are at greatest risk. Multiple surgeries also increase the risk of skin erosion. Skin erosion has the appearance of a skin color change or transparent thinning of the skin typically adjacent to the implanted hardware. Redness or new onset itching can also be a sign of skin breakdown and should be reported to your medical provider.

Wire kinking, breakage, or fraying. Symptoms related to wire damage can be subtle, intermittent, or persistent and the risk of damage increases over time. Sometimes wire damage can still allow electrical current to pass and/or electrical current to leak out into adjacent tissues causing shocks, tingling or heat sensations. In this situation, a change in posture or body position (especially the head, neck and arms) may be associated with more or less electrical current passage along the wire leading to intermittent loss of stimulation benefit or intermittent surge sensations. Symptoms associated with wire damage include:

1. Episodic or persistent tingling around the hardware or in the face, hand or foot
2. Episodic or persistent heat or warmth sensation
3. Shocks or surge sensation
4. Muscle twitching or contraction of the face, hand or foot
5. Loss of benefit

Your medical provider can check for wire damage by measuring system impedances *(an electrical measure of resistance to current flow and a measure of system integrity)*. In addition simply turning off stimulation in the office or carefully increasing the stimulation and measuring the effect are used to determine system integrity. Partial hardware damage may take time to evolve into a short circuit or open circuit that is detectable. If impedances are normal and clinical suspicion is high for a wire problem, impedances should be checked in multiple body positions such as head turning to the left and right, arm extension and flexion, standing, sitting and lying flat. An x-ray can sometimes detect a defect in the wire. Surgical replacement of the damaged wire may be needed. Wire replacement is associated with the same surgical risks as the initial implantation and therefore taken seriously.

Practical Tips: The brain (lead) wire is smaller and much more vulnerable to damage on the skull surface than the extension wire and is susceptible to damage if wearing tight straps around the head, scuba masks, scalp massage, acupuncture, or tight helmets.

Case Study. A patient reported gradual return of tremor years after DBS was implanted and a shock sensation when she reached over to turn off her light at night or while turning her head while driving. Impendence checks were initially normal but clinical suspicion was high for a problem. Persistence and patience during evaluation paid off. Repeat checks with head turning did eventually result in a measurement consistent with a broken wire. Their x-ray shows the wire damage causing her problems.

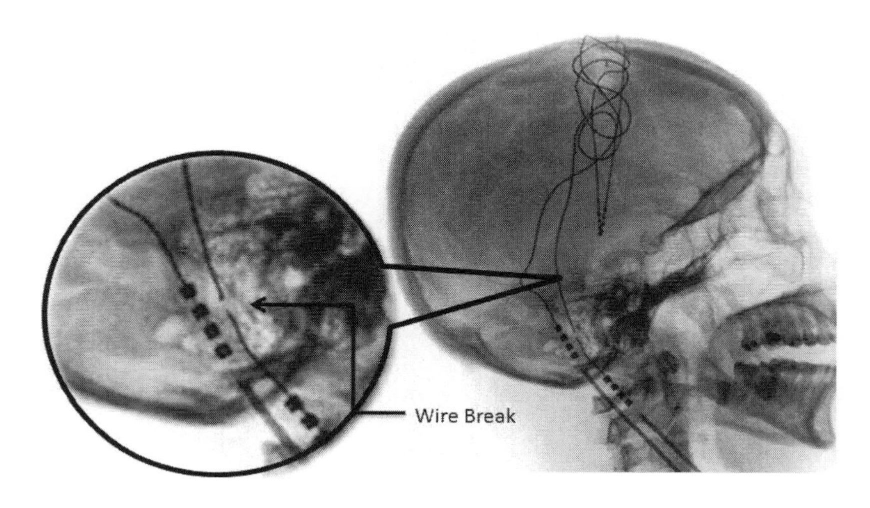

Practical Tips: Keep a diary of persistent or intermittent symptoms and the activity or situation associated with the problem. Talk to your medical provider about whether you should turn off the stimulation when experiencing shocks, heating or tingling to assess whether these symptoms quickly subside. Consider a second opinion if you are certain there is a problem that your provider is unable to detect.

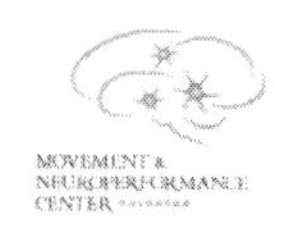

NOTES

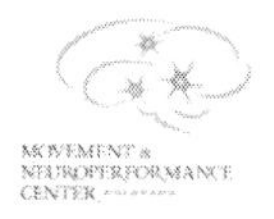

6 SAFETY

Your DBS system is essentially a brain pacemaker with wires and a power unit. This poses two general safety concerns:

- Breakage or damage of the wires, electrodes or battery
- Electrical or magnetic energy from your environment interacting with your system and potentially altering its function

At present, Medtronic, Inc. is the only FDA approved manufacturer of the device used for DBS implantation in the United States. You will be given a device identification card from Medtronic. You will find the number for Medtronic customer service on the back of your Medtronic card. The customer service department can answer questions about your device.

Damage. Damage to your system can cause a sudden or intermittent loss of therapy. Avoid damage by protecting your head and neck with an appropriate helmet during activities. Avoid situations that can cause a fall and ask for a physical therapy referral if balance is a problem. Learn how to reduce your risk of falling. Avoid aggressive massage of the head, neck and chest area as pressure and manipulation of your skin over the wires can cause wire breakage. You should also avoid acupuncture, acupressure or similar techniques when applied to your head or neck.

Travel. Make sure you have your patient programmer when you are travelling and refer to your DBS handbook (you should have received a manufacturer handbook at time of surgery) for restriction and guidance such as precautions to take while going through airports. Adding DBS to your medication list with a notation about avoiding an MRI and diathermy will remind you and others about restrictions especially when under pressure to answer questions quickly. Placing pertinent information on a medic alert bracelet alert others about your device.

DBS Safety, Environmental Considerations or Precautions. Your patient handbook explains many environmental concerns and areas or situations you should avoid. Electrical or magnetic interference can be found in many areas that include but is not limited to your home, hospital, retail centers and industrial environments. Refer to your device handbook for safety information or call customer support for up to date information.

Medical Precautions. Inform your physicians and other health care providers that you have a DBS neurostimulator implant. Certain medical procedures can cause damage to your stimulator and possibly cause you physical harm. The device company has specific guidelines and can help your physician determine the safety of a medical or surgical procedure.

Practical Tips: Your device identification card contains details about your surgery and a contact number for customer support. Keep this card with you at all times.

Warnings. At the time of this publication, body MRI is not allowed and can cause permanent injury or death if performed after DBS. Brain MRI can be done in select centers that use approved imaging protocols and equipment for some DBS devices. Failure to follow approved safety protocols can cause stroke, coma or death. Be sure to inform the technicians that you have an implanted neurostimulator.

Diathermy should never be performed. Diathermy is radiofrequency ultrasound treatment commonly used in chiropractor, dental and physical therapy offices for wound healing or sore muscles. Diathermy can cause brain damage that could result in serious injury or death.

Practical Tips: Ask your physician or clinician to contact the device company to review any safety issues before undergoing any medical or surgery procedure.

Consider purchasing a medic alert bracelet to include: Deep Brain Stimulation: Warning No MRI, Diathermy, Therapeutic Ultrasound, (include your surgeon's phone number, device company name and phone number).

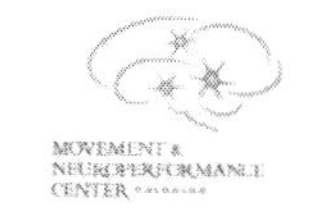

NOTES

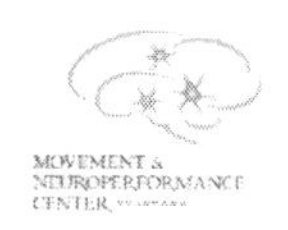

7 OPTIMAL LIVING WITH DBS

"Deep brain stimulation offers not just hope but the excitement of possibility for what the future holds. The power and potential of DBS is expanded when people are given a new outlook and can redirect life's focus. As symptoms of disease fade a new picture emerges- a brighter one with a new focus on life priorities, and personal wellbeing."
-Monique Giroux, MD

Medications

Your reliance on medications may be less as DBS improves your symptoms. This is important since many of these medications have side effects. Although less medicine means fewer side effects, you may still need some medicine to move optimally and for non-motor symptoms such as depression, anxiety, thinking or sleep problems. Therefore, it is important to remember that your primary goal for surgery is to control movement and not necessarily to stop all medication. Changes in medication doses after surgery are highly individualized and depend on the effects of stimulation, your specific movement problems and medication side effects.

Some people experience a honeymoon or microlesion effect immediately after surgery that can cause a significant improvement in symptoms. However, the microlesion effect generally wears off unexpectedly *(if you stop your medicine during this time you can experience significant difficulty when this occurs.)* The following are general guidelines regarding medication requirements after DBS.

Parkinson's disease: Your *on*-time will increase and your *off*-time will decrease as stimulation intensity is increased. As *on*-time increases, your need for medication is potentially reduced. A reduction in medication can also improve dyskinesia if you are experiencing this problem. As noted above, these changes should be done slowly in tandem with stimulation changes to get the best results from DBS. Reducing medications too soon or too much can cause you serious movement problems such as walking and balance problems. Falls can be serious since damage can occur to the DBS system. Insomnia, depression and other mood related problems can also worsen with sudden medication changes.

Tremor: Your need for tremor medication is reduced as tremor is improved. Review any medication changes with your healthcare provider since stopping suddenly can be dangerous and in some cases cause life-threatening withdrawal symptoms. This is especially important for anti-seizure medications that are used to treat tremor. Some medications used for tremor are also used to treat other problems or symptoms i.e. high blood pressure, anxiety, sleeping problems, or pain and should only be changed by your medical provider.

Dystonia: Your need for dystonia medication is reduced as dystonia is improved. Review any medication changes with your healthcare provider since suddenly stopping can be dangerous. This is especially important for anti-seizure and some anti-spasmodic medications as well as medications that also treat other problems or symptoms you may have (i.e. high blood pressure, sleeping problems, or pain.) Reducing medications too fast can worsen pain and increase risk of falling or cause life-threatening withdrawal.

Rehabilitation

Posture, walking, balance, joint pain, speech and swallowing difficulty can improve with rehabilitation both before and after surgery. Rehabilitation can help in the following ways:

- Obtain a baseline assessment prior to DBS
- Define areas that need strengthening before surgery
- Identify problems that may require rehabilitation after surgery
- Optimize your activities, performance and safety after surgery
- Treat symptoms of advanced disease such as walking and balance, speech and swallowing problems

The following worksheet is designed to help you understand the role of rehabilitation.

Rehabilitation Worksheet

Complete this to learn how rehabilitation may be helpful. Ask your neurologist for a referral to a specialist if are experiencing any of the problems noted below. Additional copies of this form can be printed from our companion website, DBSGUIDE.COM.

Physical Therapy: Specializes in physical movement such as posture, joint pain, muscle flexibility and strength, balance and mobility, and provides exercise programs.

__I need an exercise program specifically for my neurologic condition
__I am ready to increase my exercise level and activities
__I have pain that limits my activities or mobility
__I get out of breath easily when walking or feel tired most of the day
__I have trouble getting out of a chair, car or bed
__I am having trouble with walking, falling or fear of falling
__I have problems with freezing while trying to walk
__My posture is changing
__I need a walking aid such as a cane or walker
__I have exercise limitations
__My care-partner needs information how to help me move
__I have joint or muscle pain or spasms
__I have problems with coordination
__I have trouble with bladder control
__I have mobility issues that keep me from going out
__I feel dizzy when I move
__I have lost power in my legs or tire easily
__I cannot stand for very long
__I fall or have a fear of falling

Occupational Therapy: Specializes in upper body function, dexterity, self-care, medication management, daily activities, driving, transportation, and resources for independence.

__I am ready or wish to return to work
__I have problems completing tasks or organizing my day
__I need more information on how to organize my medications
__I need help or have more difficulty with dressing or bathing
__Tasks are taking longer
__I have fatigue, pain, weakness, coordination or thinking problems
__I need help with tasks, chores, work or hobbies
__I have trouble with my vision
__I have problems with freezing while trying to walk

__I am fearful of falling or fall often
__I need help with home safety
__I need help reviving my hobbies or other social interests
__I need a workplace evaluation
__I have trouble getting out of bed, chair or car
__I need help with preparing a meal
__I have trouble sleeping or moving in bed
__I am concerned about driving or have transportation problems
__I have motivation problems that affect my participation in daily activities

Speech Therapy: A comprehensive speech and voice evaluation is completed by a speech language pathologist. Therapy can help voice symptoms, swallowing difficulties, conversation and communication problems.

__I have problems swallowing food, liquid or pills
__I need to know which foods to avoid due to my swallowing problem
__I have lost more than ten pounds without trying recently
__I have excessive drooling and/or cough when I eat or drink
__I choke or worry about choking
__I have problems with my speech
__I have problems being heard or difficulty communicating
__I have word finding problems

Nutrition Consult: A registered dietician is trained to provide diet and nutritional counseling to improve nutrition, weight control, cholesterol, low and high blood pressure, leg swelling and diabetes.

__I am gaining weight (a side effect of STN stimulation) after DBS
__I am having trouble eating food due to a swallowing problem
__I am having trouble gaining weight
__My meals are interfering with my medications
__I have food sensitivities, gluten sensitivity or celiac disease
__I have diabetes or kidney disease
__I experience bowel problem or constipation

Psychology/Neuropsychology Evaluation: Specializes in the evaluation of mood changes, adjustment, anxiety and support or thinking.

__DBS has improved my symptoms but I am having trouble adjusting
__I am having trouble with my DBS and this is causing anxiety
__I have confusion, memory problems, or problems making decision

__I have more days feeling down that feeling good
__I have anxiety that interferes with my day to day activities
__I have thoughts or concerns that keep me awake at night
__My caregiver seems to be on edge, worried, or depressed

Social Work Evaluation: Provides emotional support, community resources and adjustment with an emphasis on quality of life.

__I need help finding what resources are available in your community
__I have questions regarding in home care or housing
__I am a caregiver in need of respite care
__I am interested in attending a support group for caregivers or patients
__I have interests I would like to pursue but unsure where to start
__I need help with coping
__I am having trouble communicating with others
__I am feeling overwhelmed
__I need a stronger support network

Lifestyle

Deep brain stimulation can improve quality of life. Feeling better influences your attitude about your future and your attitude plays an important role in how well you ultimately feel after DBS. This opens up an opportunity to focus on more than your disease, assess priorities and enhance your general health. Exercise, nutrition, emotional and social wellbeing are important priorities for optimal living.

Exercise. Exercise improves not only our body's physiology but also our brain's health with aging. Exercise can enhance neuroplasticity or our brain's ability to adapt, increase resiliency and function over time. For instance, researchers are now learning that exercise can not only reduce symptom progression in conditions like Parkinson's, but also improve cognitive abilities, mood and even nerve cell loss with aging.

As your motor symptoms of Parkinson's, tremor or dystonia improve so does your ability to exercise. Movement becomes easier and you are able to perform better with less frustration as rigidity, speed of movement, dexterity and coordination improves. Other changes can reduce obstacles that once limited exercise such as a more predictable response to medication, reduction in dystonic and muscular pain, improved mood, improved sleep, enhanced hopefulness about the future and reduction in medication related side effects such as sedation and fatigue.

Beginning or changing your exercise program to take advantage of your new abilities will improve fitness, stamina and general health. DBS will improve motor control but only you can improve muscle strength, stamina and fitness. Exercise will also enhance brain function to complement your restored movement. *Exercise has the potential to reduce or delay the impact of problems such as posture and imbalance that can worsen with age or disease progression.*

Keep in mind that your prior activity level will guide your exercise program. Your muscles, connective tissue, heart and lungs will need a progressive exercise routine to challenge you. In other words, your exercise routine will expand as your fitness improves. A physical therapist can help you begin or expand your exercise program to reduce injury and improve performance. Professional guidance is especially helpful if your pre-DBS symptoms limited your movement abilities. Setting and modifying goals that are within reach every four to six months will allow you advance your routine, stay motivated and experience increasing benefit over time.

Other symptoms can dictate the exercise that you do, such as apathy, depression, imbalance, arthritis, high or low blood pressure, diabetes, heart or lung disease and fatigue. Talk to your doctor or health care provider to discuss a referral to a physical therapist or an exercise physiologist to get started on a safe program. These professionals will work with you to monitor and advance your routine so that you are safe, do not get injured, stay on track, advance your routine and are successful with your program.

The following examples reinforce why exercise is important:

- Improves your agility, coordination, and stamina
- Reduces the impact of disease progression and aging- i.e. balance
- Improves mood and thinking abilities
- Reduces fatigue, improves self- confidence and body image
- Weight management (weight gain is seen after STN DBS)
- Increases bone density, joint strength and reduces joint pain
- Improves brain health
- Reduces the risk of stroke, Parkinson's and Alzheimer's disease
- Improves general health such as reduced risk of heart disease, diabetes, high blood pressure, diabetes, and even cancer

Practical Tips:

- *Work with an exercise professional for exercise guidance and progression of your routine. Set realistic goals especially if you could not exercise before DBS. Smaller goals will lead to earlier success and continue to move you forward.*
- *Do what you enjoy, be creative, add music, fun, people, pets and adventure to your routine. Include people important to you such as your family, support group members or friends.*
- *Consider cross-training to include activities that will enhance strength, flexibility, coordination, stamina, and cardiovascular fitness. Add posture, flexibility and balance exercises.*
- *Drink plenty of fluids while exercising, avoid over- heating and eat a good diet.*
- *Safety first. Balance issues, joint problems, pain, heart and lung disease, diabetes and lightheadedness are examples of problems or symptoms that require professional guidance.*

Nutrition. Nutrition is important for many reasons. Some people gain weight after DBS surgery especially with STN stimulation. The reasons for this could be many and include changes in metabolic rate, enhanced mood and appetite, increased social outings in restaurants and less energy expenditure as tremor and dyskinesia is reduced. You can combat this potential weight gain by paying attention to what you eat, monitoring your weight weekly and exercising to maintain your optimal weight.

There are more reasons to improve your nutrition beyond simply weight management. What you eat directly effects how you feel. Just as exercise helps more than just movement, your nutrition affects more than simply your weight and physique. Gaining control of your body with DBS and your stamina with exercise will require good nutrition. Even a small effort every day to make a healthy food choice, to add a new food or recipe will add a sense of accomplishment and enhanced sense of wellbeing.

We are all aware that healthy nutrition will reduce our risk of developing problems such as heart disease, diabetes, cancer, high cholesterol and high blood pressure. Nutrition can also impact mood, cognition, fatigue, and brain health. Diet fads come and go and are associated with all sorts of claims but balanced nutrition is a proven foundation for overall health. Eating a wholesome diet means eating little to no premade or processed food, packaged sweets or fast foods.

A balanced diet will supply the necessary nutrients to fight disease. The Mediterranean diet is associated with a reduced risk of heart disease, diabetes, high blood pressure and cholesterol. This diet's impact on brain health is evident by research that confirms the Mediterranean diet is associated with a lower risk of stroke, depression, dementia, and Parkinson's disease. Features of this diet:

- High in antioxidants from colorful fruits and vegetables.
- Low in inflammatory, artery clogging saturated and animal fat.
- Majority of proteins from fish, beans, grains, nuts and seeds.
- Seeds, nuts and olive oil are the primary source of healthy fats.
- Majority of carbohydrates from whole grains instead of highly processed sugary foods. These sugars slowly absorb reducing cellular and hormonal stress caused by rapid swings in blood glucose levels (this also contributes to changes in energy levels).

Practical Tips: More information on healthy eating and the link between food and brain health can be found at www.drgiroux.com.

Emotional Wellbeing. As you have learned throughout this book, feeling your best after surgery requires attention to more than just surgery and more than just movement. Your thoughts, attitude and mood will shape how you feel, how you perceive and react to the world around you.

Recognizing and treating depression and cognitive changes is very important. Depression should be treated prior to surgery and monitored thereafter. Experience confirms that depression does not always improve simply because motor symptoms are improved with DBS. Your family and friends may expect your mood to improve along with your movement symptoms after surgery but this is not always the case. Targeted treatment with medication or counseling may be required.

Talk with your doctor or healthcare provider about mood problems. Depression can be complex and can have many causes including a neurochemical imbalance, social isolation, learned negative thought patterns, learned behaviors repeated over many years, feeling of helplessness or despair and/or reaction to unmet expectations after surgery.

Depression (and mania or euphoria) can also be a side effect of stimulation. Any sudden change or worsening of your mood or behavior within a few hours or days of adjusting your stimulation should be immediately reported to your neurologist. Suicide is rare but documented after DBS. The reason(s) for this are not clear but could include untreated depression, unmet expectations and/or depression as a side effect of stimulation.

Practical Tips: A multifaceted approach to depression is best and includes counseling, medications, exercise, nutrition, good sleep and treatment of sleep apnea, stress management; focus on positive attitude and gratitude, social support and social engagement.

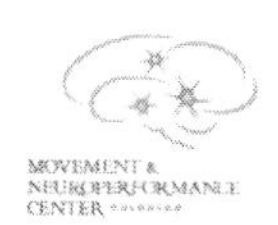

NOTES

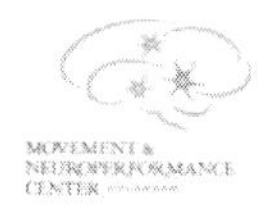

8 CAREPARTNER & FAMILY

"When I was 11 years old my mother was diagnosed with Parkinson's disease at the age of 48, and so began what was to become my life long journey as a carer/ care partner. My mother lived with PD for 37 years. I married a man who after our 10 year anniversary was diagnosed with the same disease. My husband now has PD for 40 years. Over all these years I have learned some valuable lessons. The most important is that open communication is vital, and that honesty mixed with kindness and compassion is key. It is also extremely important to take care of your own physical, mental and emotional health so that you can be fully present in the care of your loved one. Educate yourself about the disease, participate in support groups but don't go overboard and don't let PD become an obsession that robs you of all the good things you can and should still enjoy. Asking for help when you need it, without guilt, is one of the smartest things you can do. If you practice mutual respect and maintain a sense of humor, life with Parkinson's disease will be easier."

-Edna Ball; Co-Chair/Team Parkinson

This chapter is written to support the care-partner in your life; to help your family or friends better understand, cope and adjust to changes they too may experience along the way. A care-partner broadly speaking is any person in your life that is an important part of your care or assists in your healthcare and wellbeing whether family member, friend, loved one or professional healthcare assistant.

Expectations

As a care-partner you are an important part of the team, often participating in appointments, asking questions, taking notes and helping at home. Your perspective is important to share as you have insight into how things are going day after day and have a vested interest in your loved one's wellbeing. Importantly, you need to understand how DBS will impact your life together. You can cope and adjust better to change if you know what to expect after DBS surgery. You have learned the importance of expectations as DBS is not a cure.

Take a moment to review Chapters 1 paying particular attention to the information on expectations. Think about what you would like DBS to do or change for your loved one and write it down on the DBS Expectations Worksheet located in chapter 1. Compare your own expectations with those listed by your loved one and their doctor. Do these expectations match? Where are the discrepancies?

Doing this exercise together can help you understand what to expect after DBS, determine if outcomes are maximized and explore the impact of DBS on your relationship. Consider the following when reviewing your expectations for DBS:

- DBS can improve tremor. DBS can't eliminate all tremor or the effects of illness and stress on tremor.
- DBS can improve dystonia. DBS can't eliminate all dystonia or the effects of illness and stress on dystonia.
- DBS can improve Parkinson's off times, tremor, dyskinesia and rigidity. DBS cannot treat balance, speech and swallowing problems that no longer respond to dopaminergic medicine in advanced disease. DBS cannot prevent disease progression.
- DBS is not a treatment for non-movement symptoms.
- Motivation, mood, lifestyle and attitude will ultimately impact how a person with DBS feels after surgery.
- Increasing stimulation for non-responsive symptoms can lead to stimulation side effects.

Talking to your children about DBS

Children's imagination can 'run away with them', when DBS comes up in conversation. Deep brain stimulation can sound like a sci-fi movie. Talking to your children before surgery can help alleviate fears and concerns that mom or dad may not come back the same as before or that something bad will happen. Having a cursory or frank conversation depends on the age of the child and their comfort with details. A few topics for discussion include the length of time mom/dad will be in the hospital, how many days they will take to recover, what life routine will or will not change and how DBS will change symptoms.

Think about how you will communicate with your child during the day of surgery if they are not accompanying you to the hospital. The following questions were asked by children in our clinic and reflect the unique fears and concerns as seen from a child's point of view:

- How will my mom/dad look when they come home from surgery? Will their hair grow back?
- Will mom/dad be able to do the same things with me after surgery that they did before?

- How do you plug the hole (in the skull)? What kind of drill do you use? Can the drill punch through into the brain?
- Will mom be able to read my mind? Will DBS take over my mom's thoughts? Can DBS pick up radio signals so that dad can hear music?
- Will the DBS shock the brain or fry the tissue? Can the wire get rusty? Does the wire plug into a charger like a cell phone?
- Can the wire get loose and float around in the brain? How much brain tissue does DBS kill?

If you are thinking about DBS and plan to discuss the surgery with your children, consider asking your medical provider if the questions and concerns of your children can be addressed during one of your DBS appointments. Talking through fears or concerns can reduce the stress of surgery for the patient and their children.

Prepare For The Day Of Surgery

As a caregiver you will likely accompany your loved one to the hospital on the day of surgery. The following information can help ease your fears and prepare you for this day.

- Ask your surgeon for an estimate of the time for surgery to ease the anxiety of waiting and wondering.
- Bring a list of medicines and allergies to the hospital and be sure to review this list with the admission staff.
- If you can, bring someone with you to the hospital to help ease the burden of waiting alone.
- Talk to other DBS care-partners about their experience so you know what to expect.
- Know the risks of surgery. Be sure to read the surgery chapter for more information on this topic. Review the risk of problems such as confusion after surgery with your neurologist or neurosurgeon. Have a plan in place to deal with this problem before discharge.
- Pain is not generally a problem after DBS surgery and is managed with Tylenol (no aspirin, no ibuprofen containing products are used after surgery without direct conversation with the surgeon). Narcotic pain medications can bring on or worsen confusion after DBS surgery and should be used only if needed to control pain not managed with other pain medications.

- Prepare for the best and worse. What are the options if there are difficulties? This may mean an extended stay in the hospital, time away from work, inpatient rehabilitation in the hospital or transfer to a skilled nursing or rehabilitation program.
- Prepare and freeze meals in advance for the first few days you return from the hospital. Arrange time away from work; help to care for children or family members for the first few days after discharge. Although you may not need this help, it is best to be prepared in the event you do.
- Consider moving the bedroom to the first floor for a few days if balance issues are a problem.
- Get a list of 'rules' from your surgeon to help you prepare for the recovery period. For example, find out about when you can drive, return to work, exercise, and shower or use hair color.
- Take time to relax and heal each day. Even a few minutes for yourself can make a difference. Take inventory of your own feelings. Seek the help of friends, other care-partners or a counselor if you are feeling overwhelmed.

Life after DBS

As a care-partner, you may be thinking about more than just symptoms. You are thinking about how you would like life to change after DBS. When talking to care-partners about how they would like DBS to help their loved one we often hear the response, *"I just want my (husband/wife/partner) back."* There may be specific attitudes, behaviors, activities or functions that you expect will change or your loved one will now be able to do after DBS. You may also be concerned about negative changes in cognition, personality or mood after DBS. Exploring these expectations and concerns is as important as the surgical evaluation in order to be as informed as possible prior to making the decision to have surgery.

Your expectations will likely include more than just change in movement. For example, they may include not only a change in symptoms (i.e. tremor), but also activities (i.e. cooking), personal behaviors (i.e. increased motivation), impact on you (i.e. less responsibilities as a caregiver) or your relationship (i.e., more intimacy). Other examples we have heard from care-partners include wishes or expectations that your loved one will be *"able to drive, return to work, socialize or get out more, travel, exercise more, return to daily household chores or hobbies, travel, or experience increased intimacy."*

Although a return to some physical activities is likely as motor symptoms improve you can see from these examples (and perhaps your own list) that there are many unique factors or circumstances that could contribute to or even limit life change after DBS. Simply talking about these expectations will help you understand your own ideas about what you are expecting from DBS.

Depression and **apathy** (decreased motivation) deserve special mention as these symptoms/problems greatly influence your relationship and how your loved one will feel and behave after surgery. There may be a tendency to think that mood will improve and everything 'will get better' once movement improves. This is not always the case. The reason for this is that depression is sometimes a symptom of the disease and/or associated with more complex struggles in a person's life and not simply a reaction to movement difficulties. Apathy is another symptom that at times can be frustrating for care-partners. The person with apathy may struggle with the motivation to begin and complete tasks, chores and activities even if they are moving better. Depression and apathy may improve with treatment. A multi-faceted approach including a combination of medicine, counseling, exercise, diet, social activities and stress management is best. Be sure to talk with your healthcare provider about these symptoms to learn about treatment options.

Practical Tips: Being aware of mood and cognitive symptoms can help reduce frustration, realign your expectations, seek help when needed and support to maintain a positive outlook and adopt beneficial coping strategies.

Change

Change is difficult even when change is positive. After surgery your partner may be more independent with tasks and feel the freedom of new possibilities in life. Even though this is desirable, some care-partners find it difficult when roles change and the relationship becomes one of less dependence and one of more independence. Alternatively, change may not happen fast enough since some people expect a dramatic change in lifestyle after surgery. Remember that your loved one did not develop symptoms overnight. Positive change may not happen overnight and will take time.

Support

A healthy support network includes but is not limited to friends, family, your religious or spiritual community and support groups. Knowing you are not alone can be very comforting. Just having someone to talk to, knowing that you have a supportive hand when needed or can learn from others experienced with what you are now going through can make all the difference. Consider reaching out to others that are considering DBS or have already had the surgery. Sharing your experiences, lessons you have learned along the way, how you adapted to change and things you would do differently can be therapeutic for yourself as well as others. Look for a support group for caregivers in your community. Senior centers, foundations, community centers, hospitals, libraries, and religious organizations offer support groups.

Self-Care

Finally don't forget to care for yourself. Up to this point your primary focus may have been on the health and wellbeing of your loved one. The stress of surgery or a chronic disease can impact your health as the care-partner. This long-term stress can lead to anxiety, depression and even your own set of health issues. Give yourself the attention that you give others and take a moment to care for yourself. Depression is common amongst care-partners and can lead to additional health issues. Seek help if you are feeling overwhelmed, can't sleep, are more irritable, tearful, hopeless or notice change in eating habits.

Take a moment each day to pamper and self-heal. Even simple things can make a difference whether it is a massage, soothing cup of tea, or a walk in the park. Simplify life when you can. Set boundaries and say *'no'* when appropriate. Prioritize for yourself what is truly important to you at this time in your life so you do not get lost in life's hectic pace. This may mean giving up some things that you did in the past especially if they are not very important to simplify life now rather than waiting until things get difficult. Take a moment to be grateful for whomever or whatever brings value and purpose to you. The following list provides additional tips and suggestions for self- care. We urge you to find at least one thing that you can do for yourself each day.

1. Find the time and learn to relax. Simple techniques such as yoga, slow breathing, meditation or guided imagery can help.

2. Surround yourself with the healing powers of nature.

3. Relax to music.

4. Find a quiet space that is yours for self- reflection, self-care and relaxation such as a dedicated corner in a room adorned with your favorite things.

5. Try aromatherapy. Lavender and lemon balm is two essential oils found to reduce stress and improve sleep.

6. Practice mindfulness, live and be present in the moment.

7. Awaken gratitude. Think about what you are grateful for each morning upon awakening or each evening before sleep. Is there something to be grateful for today, in this moment? Did you see the sunset? Hear the laughter of a child? Consider keeping a daily gratitude journal and write down one simple thing each day that you are grateful. Writing these thoughts in a gratitude journal allows you the opportunity to read it from time to time especially on the days when life seems just a bit overwhelming.

8. Set time aside as a couple to simply talk and listen. This is especially important when dealing with expectations about surgery and potential life changes.

9. Indulge yourself in moderation and consider taking the time for simple pleasures such as chocolate, massage, videos or movie.

10. Set aside 'me-time.' Caregiving can leave you tired, zapped of energy and with little time. It is important to set aside a moment each day- even if it is just 5 minutes. Have a cup of tea, talk to a friend, keep a journal, pick up an old hobby. Find the positive and joy in life. Even simple things such as watching a comedy can take your mind away from the past or future. Do not forget your own health including yearly medical physicals and preventative health. Exercise and nutrition build up your reserves for each day.

11. **Do not lose what 'makes you- you'** and try to set aside time to continue your outside interests, passion or hobbies.

Plan Ahead

Consider how you would like to manage serious problems if they occur. Making quick decisions when under distress can only increase your stress. Planning ahead keeps you in control and more resilient to cope with unexpected or sudden changes. Life planning is an important and often neglected task. Ask your medical provider if there is a nurse or social worker that you can talk to about these issues.

Questions to consider include:

- What will you do if you can no longer take care for yourself or your loved one at home?
- Who can you call for help?
- What resources are available to you?
- Are there resources for professional caregivers when needed?

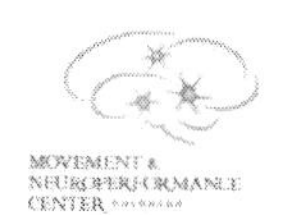

NOTES

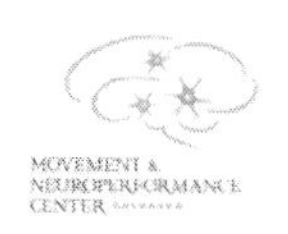

9 MYTHS

A decline in speech is a trade-off to improve symptoms.

Adjusting stimulation settings can commonly correct stimulation induced speech side effects. If speech volume or slurring cannot be improved without sacrificing benefit, the wire may not be ideally placed in the brain.

Change in walking or increased falls is always disease progression.

Mobility changes can also be a stimulation side effect or the consequence of reducing medications too fast or too much. An in depth evaluation is needed to determine the cause of worsening mobility.

DBS doesn't work for everyone.

Stimulation in the right person, appropriate brain target and adequate stimulation intensity should work and improve motor symptoms that we have experienced and witnessed across many research studies. The common causes of poor results after DBS include:

- Inappropriate diagnosis
- Misplaced electrodes
- Maladjusted stimulation settings
- Wire damage
- Unrealistic expectations

I won't gain weight after DBS.

Weight gain is well documented after bilateral subthalamic (STN) DBS. The cause is not known but is speculated to be related to a change in metabolic rate due to absence of tremor or dyskinesia. Increasing exercise may be the best way to combat weight gain after DBS.

I can go off my medication after DBS.

Medication reduction after DBS is estimated to average up to 50% for most people with STN DBS for PD, 70-100% for people with VIM DBS for tremor and substantial reductions for people with DBS for dystonia. Medication reduction depends on disease duration, type of symptoms that improve with DBS, accuracy of surgery, stimulation settings and other medical conditions.

DBS is only good for tremor.

Deep brain stimulation is known to improve more than just tremor. Stiffness, slowness, shuffling, dystonia, extend the time Parkinson's medications are working, reduce dyskinesia, reduce pain from dystonia, and continues to work unless the stimulation is turned off.

Anyone can adjust my stimulation.

Applying stimulation to the brain should be done by a medical provider that is board certified and has a medical license to administer a medical treatment. The response to stimulation that occurs while adjusting stimulation should be under the direct supervision of the person responsible for the care and outcome for the patient. Stimulation adjustments should not be performed by non-medical personnel for your safety and overall well-being.

DBS is a treatment of *'last resort.'*

Deep brain stimulation is recommended before Parkinson's disease reaches advanced stages and/or before medication side effects become a serious problem. DBS will be less effective in advance stages due to the many symptoms at this stage that are not responsive to medicine and are therefore not responsive to DBS.

Worsening symptoms are always disease progression.

As reviewed in chapters four and five, stimulation can mimic symptoms of disease progression, worsen movement, speech and swallowing and lead to instability and falls. Any worsening of symptoms should be investigated, especially when symptoms that respond well to stimulation worsen.

Any surgeon can put in DBS hardware.

The day you spend in the operating room with the surgeon is ***the first day of the rest of your life*** with DBS. Choose a surgeon that works closely with a team experienced in DBS care and long-term management. Getting to surgery fast is not always best. Surgical risk must be identified and this risk reduced (this can take time and further evaluation) since complications can cause permanent disability or death. Be wary of surgeons or teams that criticize proven techniques, make unbelievable claims that are too good to be true, down play the risks of surgery or unable to provide you with details about their rate of infection, rate of hemorrhage or number of reoperations due to their lead positioning. All surgeons will experience complications as complications are inherent with any surgery. Beware of teams that have little understanding of the potential harm that can occur when DBS fails to meet your expectations or worse, minimize the risk of brain surgery.

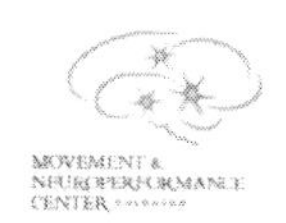

NOTES

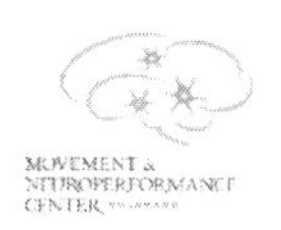

10 FREQUENTLY ASKED QUESTIONS

WHAT IS DEEP BRAIN STIMULATION?

Deep Brain Stimulation is a surgical therapy for Parkinson's disease, dystonia or tremor. The therapy involves the implantation of tiny wires into specific areas of the brain. The wires connect to a small battery (neurostimulator) that is placed under the collarbone. The neurostimulator is similar to a heart pacemaker. Once activated, the neurostimulator sends continuous electrical impulses to the specific brain region known to improve symptoms.

HOW DOES DBS WORK?

How electrical current improves symptoms is still unknown. When stimulation is turned off, the effect of stimulation disappears and symptoms typically return.

IS DBS SURGERY PAINFUL?

Local anesthesia is used prior to putting on the head frame and other forms of sedation are available to lessen the awareness and anxiety during preparation or when undergoing the brain MRI or CT scan. Sedation is commonly used during the burr hole preparation however, each surgeon will have a preference for how little or how much sedation during the surgery. There is mild to moderate pain from the head frame pins and additional local anesthesia can reduce the discomfort during and after the procedure. Ice can be very helpful for the scalp to lessen any residual pain from the head frame pins or fiducial screws. Lastly, people usually report pain in the upper chest after the neurostimulator battery is implanted that lasts until the area has healed. Most people require only a mild pain reliever (must be approved by surgeon) during the final healing stages.

HOW DO I KNOW IF I AM A GOOD CANDIDATE FOR DBS?

Neurologists who have training in movement disorders and DBS can determine if DBS is a good choice for you. The evaluation for DBS involves several appointments that determine if DBS will improve your symptoms and identify risks. You can read about the full details about this evaluation in chapter 2.

WHICH SYMPTOMS TYPICALLY BENEFIT FROM STIMULATION?
Parkinson's symptoms that respond to stimulation include tremor, stiffness, slowness and shuffling gait. DBS increases the amount of time that PD medicines last (reduced *off*-time). People with tremor will typically experience an average of 70% reduction in tremor, depending on the type and location of tremor. Dystonia is a very complex condition with complex symptoms. In some cases, dystonic posturing, pain and dystonic tremor can respond very well to stimulation.

IS DBS A CURE?
No, DBS is not a cure. It is a treatment that works to help specific symptoms related to PD, tremor and dystonia.

SHOULD I HAVE DBS ON ONE SIDE OF THE BRAIN OR BOTH SIDES?
DBS on one side of the brain improves symptoms on the opposite side of the body. Implanting the wires on both sides will offer the best results and overall improvement in motor function if patients have symptoms on both sides of the body. For patients whose symptoms are mainly affecting one side of the body, DBS surgery on the opposite side of the brain may be sufficient.

WILL I BE ABLE TO STOP TAKING MY MEDICATIONS AFTER I HAVE DBS?
DBS is not a substitute for medications. After the DBS system has been adjusted, your neurologist will likely lower medication doses based on the results of stimulation. Although most patients will need to remain on some medications after DBS surgery, many will be able to lower their medications. The total dose needed after DBS surgery is very difficult to predict. Most Parkinson patients will not be able to stop medicine completely. Patients with tremor predominant disease and no fluctuations are more likely to experience a greater decrease in medicine. People with dystonia and essential tremor may be able to reduce or stop

WHAT IF DBS DOESN'T WORK?
In the appropriate selected person, DBS stimulation is effective in improving the symptoms and problems noted in this book. If DBS doesn't work or symptoms worsen right after surgery, the cause should be investigated. Wires can be unknowingly damaged during the surgery or the electrodes may not be in the ideal location. If you have not improved within six months of surgery, discuss this with your doctor. For the best possible results, choose a DBS team with a neurosurgeon, movement disorders

neurologist, and healthcare team that are trained and experienced in DBS therapy. Review chapter 5 for more information.

ARE THERE ACTIVITIES THAT I NEED TO AVOID OR CANNOT DO AFTER HAVING DBS SURGERY?
Generally you will return to normal daily functions within a few weeks of DBS surgery. Always check with your neurologist and/or surgeon for specific guidelines. As a general rule, you will need to avoid neck manipulation or traction, massage, or acupuncture near the implanted hardware device, arc welding, body MRI, diathermy ultrasound and high intensity electromagnetic environments.

ARE THERE ELECTRICAL DEVICES IN MY HOME OR COMMUNITY THAT I SHOULD AVOID?
Most household electrical devices are safe to use, including microwaves, radios, and computers. Some high power machinery can be dangerous such as that used for electric arc-welders. Consult with your DBS medical provider or Medtronic customer support for advice if you use power tools or large machinery.

IF A CURE OR NEW TREATMENT FOR PD IS FOUND, CAN I HAVE THE DBS SYSTEM REMOVED?
Yes. DBS is reversible. The implanted wires and neurostimulator can be removed without damaging the brain.

CAN I EXERCISE AFTER HAVING DBS? Most people return to exercise within four to six weeks after DBS surgery incisions have completely healed. Full contact sports or aggressive exercise can increase the risk of hardware damage. Exercise is important for your health, neuroplasticity and to offset weight gain. Consult with your DBS team if you have any concerns or questions about your activities.

WILL MY INSURANCE PAY FOR MY DBS SURGERY?
Since DBS is approved by the FDA, many insurance payers cover the costs of DBS surgery and programming adjustments.

HOW LONG WILL THE BATTERY LAST?
The neurostimulator battery typically lasts between two and five years. Battery life varies depending on the intensity of your stimulation settings. If battery power is lost, your symptoms will likely worsen and more medication may be needed until the neurostimulator is replaced. Your neurologist or DBS programmer will periodically check the battery and inform you when the neurostimulator should be replaced. Your patient

programmer will allow you to track your battery status at home. The neurostimulator battery is replaced as an outpatient surgical procedure.

CAN DBS STOP WORKING SUDDENLY AFTER WORKING FOR SEVERAL MONTHS OR YEARS?

Yes. Common reasons for loss of therapy are depleted battery power or the device is damaged. For example, there could be a break in the wire. If your symptoms suddenly worsen, contact your DBS team immediately.

WILL I BE ASLEEP DURING DBS SURGERY?

During the implantation of the wire into the brain, the surgeon may or may not require that you be awake. If your symptoms need to be evaluated during surgery, you will be awake and asked questions about how you feel and your symptoms will be examined while the stimulation is tested. You may experience both a reduction in symptoms and brief sensations as the surgeon activates stimulation to measure both benefit and side effects to confirm adequate placement of the wire. You are typically asleep for the battery implantation.

WHAT ARE THE COMPLICATIONS OF DBS SURGERY?

Bleeding in the brain is the most concerning complication of DBS surgery. Seizures rarely occur during or after wire implantation. Infection of the skin or the implanted hardware is also a possible complication of surgery. Other complications include muscle weakness, speech changes, walking or balance problems, word finding problems and confusion. When testing the stimulation, reversible side effects may include slurred speech, dizziness, tingling, lightheadedness, vision changes or muscle contraction. Although rare, as in any surgery, death can occur as a consequence of surgery. Risks can be minimized with a thorough evaluation and care by an experienced DBS team. Your surgeon will discuss the risks and complications of DBS surgery.

HOW WELL DOES DBS WORK?

DBS is as good as medicine for people with Parkinson's essentially expanding the medicine on-time and reducing medicine off time. An exception is the symptom of tremor. DBS helps Parkinson's tremor even when medication does not. Other types of tremor, such as Essential tremor, can be reduced on average of 70% with benefit sustained over many years. DBS works well for dystonia in carefully selected individuals. Your outcome to stimulation depends on an accurate evaluation, proper electrode placement, intact DBS hardware, and appropriate DBS adjustment and medication dosage.

HOW LONG WILL DBS WORK?
DBS is known to work for over a decade. Research has confirmed DBS keeps working to improve the same symptoms that improved initially with DBS. However, the stimulation must be properly adjusted over the years and the batteries must be replaced before depleting for DBS to provide relief of symptoms. When the neurostimulator is turned off, symptoms typically return in a short period of time. Parkinson's disease does progress and symptom progression continues. Review with your neurologist typical patterns of progression after DBS surgery.

SHOULD I TURN OFF THE STIMULATION?
Stimulation should be on at all times if you have Parkinson's disease or dystonia. Some people with Essential tremor turn off the stimulator at night. Do not turn off your stimulator unless you have discussed this with your physician.

DOES DBS HAVE AN ADVANTAGE OVER OTHER TYPES OF BRAIN SURGERY?
DBS is considered an advance in surgical therapy for the treatment of Parkinson's, tremor and dystonia. DBS has several benefits over lesion surgery which permanently destroys brain areas (thalamotomy including ultrasound, gamma knife and pallidotomy). Lesion therapies are permanent, cannot be reversed and are not adjustable. DBS is reversible and the hardware can be removed if needed without causing trauma to the brain. DBS therapy is adjustable and any side effects from stimulation are reversible by changing the stimulation parameters. DBS hardware can be removed and replaced if the wire location is inadequate.

WHAT ARE THE RESTRICTIONS AFTER SURGERY?
Your surgeon's office will provide any necessary restrictions. Ask your surgeon about driving or lifting heavy weight or strenuous exercise or activity. You should not immerge yourself in a soaking tub until your incisions are completely healed.

WHO WILL TAKE CARE OF MY INCISIONS?
Your surgeon will remove any staples or sutures that remain after you leave the hospital. Remember, the skin is held together by staples or sutures and you should not remove them yourself. Ask the surgeon to examine any visible suture tips. Do not remove your sutures or pick at any protruding suture tips or knots.

WHAT ARE THE GENERAL RECOMMENDATIONS TO PREVENT DAMAGE TO MY DBS DEVICE?

Be sure that you understand where the different components of your DBS system are located on your body to help you reduce the risk of hardware damage. Ask your doctor to show you the actual hardware that will be implanted. Trauma near or over the device can damage the wires or battery. Picking or fiddling with the wires or battery can damage the system. A fall or hit to the head can also cause the wire to break. If you have concerns the hardware may be damaged, see your DBS medical provider for a system checkup. Avoid massage or acupuncture near the wires including the skull since you may not be able to feel where the wires are coiled on your skull.

SHOULD I OBTAIN A MEDICAL ALERT BRACELET OR NECKLACE?

This is recommended for your safety. The alert can include: Warning Deep Brain Stimulation, No MRI, No Diathermy, No therapeutic ultrasound. Also include your physician's name and Medtronic's phone number.

ARE THERE ANY CONCERNS FOR SUN EXPOSURE?

Protect the skin around your incisions from excessive sun exposure. Sunburn can damage your skin which can lead to erosion or skin infection. See your neurosurgeon for guidance if your surgeon or dermatologist recommends removal of skin cancer on the scalp since the wires lie under the scalp.

WHEN CAN I RESUME DRIVING AFTER DBS SURGERY?

Your surgeon will decide when you can resume driving. If you had a seizure during or after the surgery, your driving restriction may be prolonged.

CAN I HAVE ELECTROLYSIS?

Electrolysis should not be used over the implanted device.

WHO WILL INFORM MY OTHER PHYSICIANS THAT I HAVE HAD DBS SURGERY?

You should remind all your physicians and medical providers that you have DBS especially dentists, chiropractors, therapists, surgeons and dermatologists.

ARE THERE SPECIAL PRECAUTIONS FOR MEDICAL TESTS OR THERAPIES?

Body MRI (any body part other than the brain) is not allowed at this time. Body MRI can cause brain damage or death. Brain MRI can be done if the MRI scanning meets Medtronic's safety protocol with the correct equipment. Few centers have this MRI compatible equipment. Speak with your DBS providers before having any type of MRI. If a brain MRI is needed, the DBS system will need to be checked and then turned off. Damaged hardware may exclude the person from having a brain MRI. The DBS neurostimulator should be turned off for CT scans and during any type of surgery. Regular X-rays are safe without restrictions. Your medical provider should inquire with Medtronic about safety measures necessary during any surgery.

CAN I HAVE DIATHERMY ULTRASOUND TREATMENT?
Diathermy should never be used after DBS. Use of diathermy can cause severe brain injury or death. Diathermy is an electrically induced heat (high-frequency electromagnetic waves) therapy commonly used to treat an injury or wound.

ARE THERE ANY LIMITATIONS FOR IMPLANTED PACEMAKERS OR DEFIBRILLATORS BEFORE OR AFTER DBS?
Implanted heart devices can be used with DBS, however the DBS neurostimulator will require specific stimulation settings if the person also has a heart medical device. Your medical provider can contact Medtronic for specific recommendations and compatibility information.

DOES TRANSCUTANEOUS ELECTRICAL NERVE STIMULATION (TENS) INTERFERE WITH MY DBS?
TENS is commonly used for muscle injuries to reduce pain. TENS may or may not be appropriate and should be used with caution and only after Medtronic has been consulted by your medical or rehabilitation provider. The location of the TENS electrode pads must be kept away from your system and these specific instructions must be discussed with Medtronic prior to use.

DO MAGNETS INTERFERE WITH MY DBS?
Magnetic devices can interfere with the implanted hardware and patient programming device (especially older batteries). It is best to avoid strong magnetic devices if at all possible to minimize any potential interference. Consult with Medtronic for specific restrictions.

WHAT IF I NEED ADDITIONAL MEDICAL DEVICES OR PROCEDURES AFTER DBS IS IMPLANTED?
Medtronic customer support can provide you medical provider with the most up-to-date safety information and compatibility with other devices and treatment. This includes lithotripsy for kidney stones, radiation therapy, heart and other pacemakers and surgery.

WHAT SHOULD I DO AT THE AIRPORT OR OTHER SECURITY SCANNERS?
Follow the guidelines per your DBS physician. Be sure to have your Medtronic ID card with you when you are traveling. You will typically receive the ID card within three to four weeks after your surgery.

CAN I ARC WELD?
No, arch welding is currently not recommended by Medtronic and should be avoided.

SHOULD I AVOID MY PET AFTER DBS SURGERY?
Avoid direct skin contact with your pets near your incisions until the skin is completely healed. Wash your hands after handling any animal to reduce risk of infection. A general and proactive step is to avoid sleeping with your pet until all incisions are completely healed.

CAN I SAFELY USE INDUSTRIAL TYPE EQUIPMENT?
Industrial equipment may emit strong electromagnetic levels. Consult with the equipment manufacturer whether medical devices can be safely used near the industrial equipment. Consult with Medtronic customer service if the equipment manufacturer is uncertain about the safety of you and your implanted hardware. Always check your neurostimulator if you have been exposed to high energy electromagnetic fields.

CAN I CONTINUE TO SCUBA DIVE, SKYDIVE, WIND SURF, OCEAN SURF, SKI, HIKE OR GO TO HIGH ALTITUDE?
Medtronic does not recommend diving below 10 meters. High impact sports can result in damage to the hardware. High altitude should not affect the neurostimulator but may impact your judgment about safety. Falling, sudden jerks, twists can damage your implanted hardware. Talk to your DBS team prior to any of these activities.

WHERE CAN I LEARN MORE ABOUT DBS?
You will receive a handbook from Medtronic that will review many of the questions noted above. Medtronic customer support is available to answer your questions. Medtronic also provides online resources.

LEARN MORE ABOUT THESE TOPICS AND MORE AT
www.dbsprogramming.com.

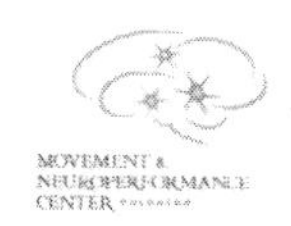

NOTES

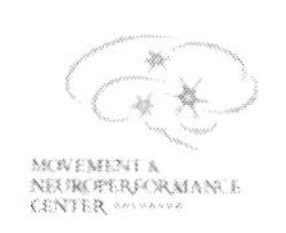

11 RESOURCES

WEBSITE: DBSGUIDE.COM

The following forms are available for you to download, print and complete to optimize your medical care.

1. Expectation & Symptom Worksheet
2. Be Prepared: Ask Questions before DBS
3. Rehabilitation Worksheet
4. Caregiver Self-Care Guide
5. Troubleshooting Article: Retrospective Review of Factors Leading to Dissatisfaction with STN DBS during Long-term Management.

BLOG: WWW.DBSPROGRAMMER.COM

DBSProgrammer.com contains important information about DBS by blogger Sierra Farris.

BLOG: WWW.DRGIROUX.COM

DrGiroux.com. Dr. Giroux's blog contains helpful tips to support better living with dystonia, tremor and Parkinson's disease from medication, lifestyle to wellness.

NORTHWEST PARKINSON'S FOUNDATION

www.nwpf.org. The NWPF supports the Parkinson's community in the Northwest and is an example of the power of collaboration when organizations, professionals and community work together.

DAVIS PHINNEY FOUNDATION

www.davisphinneyfoundation.org. The Davis Phinney Foundation embraces the champion attitude and inspiration of founder Davis Phinney to live you best today. Our partner in publishing the Every Victory Counts. Essential information and inspiration for a lifetime of wellness with Parkinson's disease.

INTERNATIONAL ESSENTIAL TREMOR FOUNDATION

www.essentialtremor.org. Provides education, services and support.

DYSTONIA MEDICAL RESEARCH FOUDATION
www.dystonia-foundation.org. Active in research, awareness and support.

MEDTRONIC
Online support is found at www.medtronicdbs.com. Patient services can be reached at 1-800-510-6735. Keep your device information current (1-800-551-5544).

About the Authors

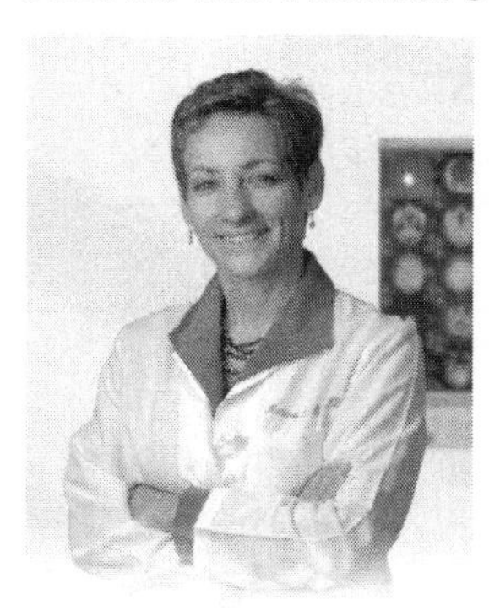

Monique Giroux, MD embraces a holistic approach includes medical, surgical, rehabilitative and integrative therapies with a particular focus on life-style for brain health. Dr. Giroux completed two years of fellowship training in movement disorders and DBS in 1996 at Emory University in Atlanta Georgia. Dr. Giroux is the only U.S. Neurologist to complete fellowship training in Movement Disorders and Integrative Medicine. She is medical director of Swedish Medical Center Movement Disorders and DBS program in Englewood, CO, medical faculty for National Parkinson's Foundation's National Allied Team Training , and medical director of the Northwest Parkinson's Foundation. She has experience and leadership in interdisciplinary care, extensive training in DBS management, Botox therapies, and mindfulness based therapies. Giroux and Sierra Farris have been working as a team to advance DBS care since 2000.

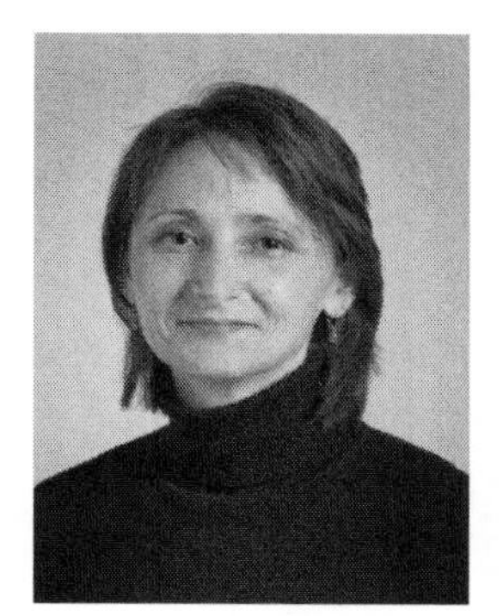

Sierra Farris, MA, MPAS, PA-C is a board certified Physician Assistant since 1998 with master's degrees in both Clinical Neurology and Bioethics. She has extensive experience in the medical, surgical and rehabilitative treatment of individuals with movement disorders and has treated over 1000 people with deep brain stimulation including international patients. Sierra developed and manages an intensive troubleshooting clinic for people with unsatisfactory results from DBS. Sierra is one of a few national DBS programming instructors serving as medical faculty for Medtronic since 2004 that includes advanced troubleshooting seminars. Sierra's research and publications focus on improving the outcomes for people living with DBS. Sierra's background as a certified Clinical Exercise Specialist by the American College of Sports Medicine adds to her repertoire to counsel patients about exercise strategies for optimal health.

Other Patient Books or Chapters by the Authors

Every Victory Counts. Essential information and inspiration for a lifetime of wellness with Parkinson's disease. Coauthored by Dr. Giroux and Sierra Farris. The manual is a comprehensive self-care guide focused on inspiration, and personal empowerment for all people wanting to take control of life with PD. Published by the Davis Phinney Foundation.

More Than a Mountain. Dr. Giroux and Sierra Farris provided a chapter about their personal experience climbing a high altitude mountain with their patients. The book chronicles the first Parkinson's and Multiple Sclerosis expedition to Mt Kilimanjaro for which Dr. Giroux and Sierra served as medical support team. The climber's stories filled with inspiration, fears, dreams, courage and compassion remind us all to redefine the possible.

Life with a Battery Operated Brain - A Patient's Guide to Deep Brain Stimulation Surgery for Parkinson's Disease. Authored by Jackie Hunt Christensen. Sierra Farris is a contributing author on the topic of technical aspects of deep brain stimulation. Jackie provides the patient perspective into a high tech brain surgery. These insights are a valuable resource for any person considering DBS.

Navigating Life with Parkinson's Disease. Sierra Farris is a contributing author on the topic of deep brain stimulation. A marvelous guide for anyone affected by Parkinson's disease including patients, caregivers, family members, and friends. Published as part of the American Academy of Neurology Now book series.

Made in the USA
San Bernardino, CA
11 November 2014